The Extracellular Matrix in Health and Disease

Fraser Smith

The Extracellular Matrix in Health and Disease

Naturopathic Approaches to Improve Structure and Function

Springer

Fraser Smith
Clinical Sciences; Naturopathic Medicine
National University of Health Sciences
Lombard, IL, USA

ISBN 978-3-031-94464-2 ISBN 978-3-031-94465-9 (eBook)
https://doi.org/10.1007/978-3-031-94465-9

This Springer imprint is published by the registered company Springer Nature Switzerland AG
The registered company address is: Gewerbestrasse 11, 6330 Cham, Switzerland

I dedicate this book to my mother, the late Ethel Smith who passed away at the age of 96 during the completion of this manuscript. Her life of love and service will always inspire me. My Mom, and Dad, encouraged me to become a naturopathic doctor and to pursue my career since graduating. In the past years, my Mom always had copies of my books to show visitors. My parents put great value on authorship and instilled the respect for knowledge, and books, in me as a child. And as an adult, they were always there to cheer me on.

Acknowledgments

This book is a needed bridge between the dynamic and vital field of naturopathic medicine, and the rapidly growing field of research into the extracellular matrix. As always, I wish to thank my colleagues at the National University of Health Sciences, which is my academic home. I also thank my students, with whom I discuss these concepts and which motivates me to learn more.

This book would not be possible without the many scientists who have created this knowledge and are expanding and refining it. I also thank my mentors: Dr. Paul Saunders, Dr. Pamela Snider, Dr. Jared Zeff, and Dr. Louise Edwards. And most importantly, thank you to my family who share me with these kinds of projects—without the encouragement of my wife, Dr. Debra Orr—this book would never have come to fruition. A special thanks to Channing Smith for the illustration, and Dexter Smith for making me get outside and exercise—addressing my own requirements for health.

Contents

1 The Interconnected Body: The Structure of the Extracellular Matrix and Its Role

There is a system of the body that is vastly more pervasive than even the circulatory system. It is the precondition of cellular viability. It acts as a connection between cells and as a meta-system of communication throughout the body. Its normal structure and function support cells in their normal state, and its dysfunction precedes and, in some ways, defines the extent of cellular pathology [1, 2]. This system is the extracellular matrix (ECM).

In spite of the role of the ECM as a sort of prime mover toward homeostasis in the human body, there remains a lack of focused work on therapeutic measures to restore health by improving the ECM (Fig. 1.1). This situation is changing as scientific research into how therapies: plant extract, physical, energetic, and nutritional can alter the ECM for the better in precise ways that relate to health and disease. The research into this system was begun in the twentieth century and has accelerated in the twenty-first century.

Even if the ECM was a zone of the body where important events, such as toxin trappage or microbial invasion occurred, it would warrant serious attention for medical and therapeutic purposes. But the ECM is much more than this. Due to its close communication, and in fact, physical connection with cells and their nuclei, the ECM is an influence on genetic expression. It works in tandem with cells, and it is a full participant in both homeostasis and the dysfunctions that lead to disease states.

F. Smith, *The Extracellular Matrix in Health and Disease*,
https://doi.org/10.1007/978-3-031-94465-9_1

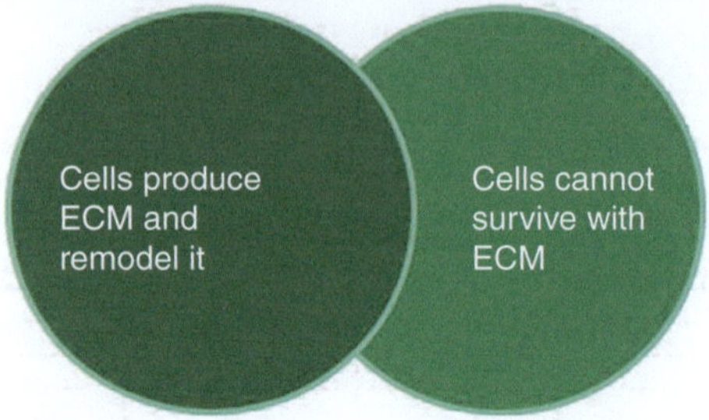

Fig. 1.1 ECM and cell

The changes in the ECM are visible and well documented in states such as aging, inflammation, injury, and cancer. ECM degradation precedes and, to some extent, defines various pathologies [3, 4]. Moreover, as people age, their ECM becomes less organized and functional. With time, oxidative stress, weakness, rigidity due to collagen cross-linking, and senescent behavior of matrix dwelling cells become a major burden on the ECM. The breakdown of the ECM is coincident with various breakdowns in the lifespan of an individual.

In this textbook, we'll examine some of the salient features of the extracellular matrix. This includes the various molecules that compose it and the cells that inhabit it. This includes proteins such as collagen, various proteoglycans, and growth factors that are stored within vesicles or directly bound to proteoglycans. The cells of the ECM include fibroblasts, macrophages, and other white blood cells that might visit depending on local events. Stem cells in various tissues tend to cluster in certain areas adjacent to ECM and form a niche. The discussion will also include some of the many growth, nutritional, eliminative, and regulatory functions of the ECM. These have been well described in great detail in the past several decades of intensive research in this area. This summary of functions is presented with an emphasis on the ways in which cellular health is dependent on the ECM. This vital network in many ways determines the *terrain* in which the organism and its specific cellular types can operate, or, can break down.

This textbook will then present a naturopathic model of using supportive and corrective therapies whose use is informed by an analysis of the various *levels of dysfunction* in a given organ or organism. This is highly related to an understanding of how naturopathic therapies can influence the extracellular matrix. On this basis, we'll proceed to look at seven levels of dysfunction in an organ or tissue, beginning with more superficial and easily reversible hypofunction, to progressive levels of dysregulation, inflammation, fibrosis, and organ failure. For each of these levels, we will discuss how the ECM is involved in the disease and dysfunction process, what ECM changes precede the dysfunction, and how ECM disruption defines the extent of dysfunction. The preventive and corrective approaches that naturopathic medicine could offer are incorporated into this discussion.

These levels of dysfunction were described in the previous textbook, "Naturopathic Medicine, A Comprehensive Guide," published by Springer in 2022 [5]. They are not usually not fixed or permanent states, and not actual diagnoses (although they denote similar kinds of diagnoses). This type of hierarchy is useful for a naturopathic medicine approach. This system of medicine seeks to remove the disturbances to health, fortify the self-healing mechanisms, and add nontoxic supplemental biochemical and whole person support. It absolutely entails the intelligent, and compassionate, use of allopathic therapies in many situations. That is to say, naturopathic medicine is a primary care method that is adaptable to virtually all situations, but it is not an alternative to or exclusive of standard medical care (Fig. 1.2).

This leads to a look at a rapidly accumulating and fascinating area of discovery about the extracellular matrix and neoplasia. The *tumor microenvironment* is highly determinant of the success of cancer cells in dividing, invading, and disseminating. Remarkably, that microenvironment is to a large extent created by cancer cells, which seize control of the ECM, including local fibroblasts and macrophages.

The implications of the study of this substrate of cellular life, the extracellular matrix, for naturopathic medicine are of high importance. The alternation of the micro-physiology of organs and issues, the re-regulation of local systems of lymph, immune,

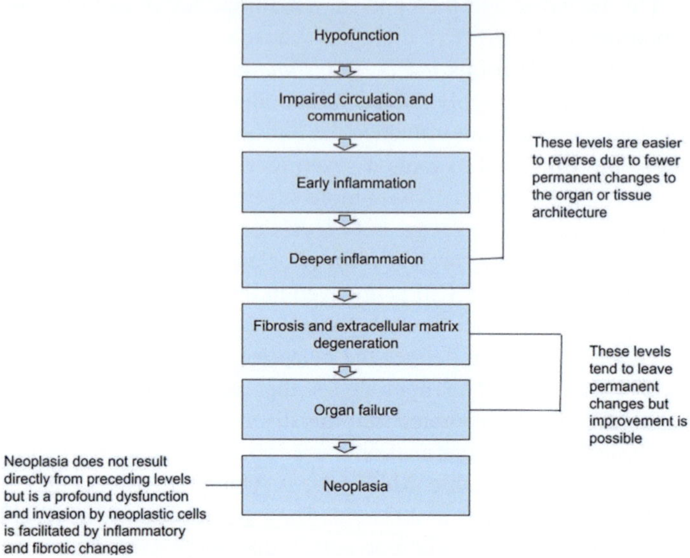

Fig. 1.2 Levels of dysfunction

and nutritive function, the expression of reparative or pro-survival genes, the architectural normalization of microstructures, and the inhibition of destructive processes are all properly the province of naturopathic medicine. In many ways, it is the main business of naturopathic medicine to create the conditions for health.

Exciting findings in biomedical research are unveiling specific disease mechanisms and prospective repair pathways. While our insight into ECM function in precise areas of a patient at one moment in time is limited, and our ability to even understand how the organism-wide ECM communicates is still developing, we can approach the ECM in some eminently practical ways. One is that we have quite a bit of knowledge about its normal structure and function. Second is that the changes to ECM in various disease states are well documented. The third is that the impact of natural therapies on the ECM is already well documented and continually building in depth and clarity.

It is the hope of this author that this book encourages physicians, researchers, and students to further explore the ECM. Even as the convergence of molecular biology techniques and accumulation of biochemical and genetic information allows us to pinpoint specific problems, a comprehensive understanding of the ECM allows us to see the human organism working as a highly integrated system. That understanding opens the door for treatments that reintegrate and restore the structure and function of the human body at a most fundamental level.

References

1. Karamanos NK, Theocharis AD, Piperigkou Z, Manou D, Passi A, Skandalis SS, et al. A guide to the composition and functions of the extracellular matrix. The. FEBS J. 2021;288(24):6850.
2. Marastoni S, Ligresti G, Lorenzon E, Colombatti A, Mongiat M. Extracellular matrix: a matter of life and death. Connect Tissue Res. 2008;49(3–4):203–6.
3. Iozzo RV, Gubbiotti MA. Extracellular matrix: the driving force of mammalian diseases. Matrix Biol. 2018;71:1–9.
4. Theocharis AD, Manou D, Karamanos NK. The extracellular matrix as a multitasking player in disease. FEBS J. 2019;286(15):2830–69.
5. Smith F. Naturopathic medicine. Cham: Springer; 2022.

Molecules of the Extracellular Matrix: Types of Extracellular Matrix Molecules and Their Roles

2

The extracellular matrix (ECM) has some recurring molecular features, but their array, composition, and configuration vary locally. There are various proteins, as well as proteoglycans (PGs) (which denotes a carbohydrate moiety on a protein) and water. There are structural proteins such as collagens and the proteoglycans tend to retain water which gives the ECM a gel-like composition. Proteoglycans are a subclass of glycoproteins (Table 2.1) which have both structural functions and effects on cell replication and motility.

Table 2.1 Glycoproteins examples

Collagens	Elastins	Tenascins	Fibronectin	Laminin
Structural network and basement membrane stability Communication	Viscoelastic properties of the ECM	Bind actin filaments in the cell to integrin	Connect integrin to extracellular proteins	Basement membrane structure and cell motility

F. Smith, *The Extracellular Matrix in Health and Disease*,
https://doi.org/10.1007/978-3-031-94465-9_2

Proteoglycans

Proteoglycans are protein-based structures that have an attached glycosaminoglycan.

Glucosaminoglycans (GAGs), chains of repeating disaccharides, include amino sugars. GAGs are components of proteoglycans and vary depending on the tissue they compose. These include:

- Heparin sulfate
- Chondroitin sulfate
- Keratin sulfate
- Dermatan sulfate

PGs (Table 2.2) attract water and help keep the ECM in a hydrated gel state, which allows for easier chemical reactions, resistance to compression and stretch, and overall fullness of structure of the body's tissues. PGs also bind vesicles which contain growth factors such as epithelial growth factor (EGF), vascular endothelial growth factor (VEGF), and platelet-derived growth factor (VEGF). Vesicles also contain microRNA which impacts the translation of messenger RNA by binding to it and blocking it [1–3].

Heparin sulfate can also be found free or non-covalently bound to proteins.

Table 2.2 Proteoglycan examples of the ECM

Type	Examples	Function	Glycosaminoglycan attached
Cell membrane	Beta-glycan	Receptor for TGFBR3	Chondroitin sulfate, heparin sulfate
Pericellular–basement membrane	Perlecan	Polarization of basement membrane Epithelial cells	Heparin sulfate
Pericellular–hyaluronate binding	Aggrecan	Helps cartilage withstand stress—load bearing	Chondroitin sulfate, keratin sulfate

(continued)

Table 2.2 (continued)

Type	Examples	Function	Glycosaminoglycan attached
Extracellular–small lecuring rich proteoglycans (SLRP)	Biglycan	Collagen stability and cell migration	Chondroitin sulfate
SLRP	Decorin	Collagen stability and cell migration	Dermatan sulfate
SLRP	Fibromodulin	Stabilize fibrillar networks	Keratan sulfate
SLRP	Osteoglycin	Bone formation and muscle–bone linkages	Keratan sulfate
SLRP	Chondroadherin	Connects chondrocytes, fibroblasts, and osteoblasts in cartilage	Chondroitin sulfate
SLRP	Podocan	Collagen binding may limit cell migration	Keratan sulfate
SPOCK gene released	Testican	Under investigation	Chondroitin sulfate

Modified from Iozzo and Schaefer [3]

Small Leucine-Rich Proteoglycans (SLRPs)

This is a large grouping of proteoglycans, with at least 18 types. SLRPs are bound to collagen and have a role in the production of collagen fibrils. They also bind to various growth factors, as well as cytokines. SLRP can also bind to cell surface receptors.

Examples include:

Versican

Veriscan is a high molecular weight sodium hyaluronic acid. It is found throughout the body including joint tissue and the heart. It is a major attractant to water and hydrates tissues.

Decorin and Biglycan

These SLRPs are involved in collagen stability and also cell adhesion and migration. They also can interact with TGF-β. They may, in some tissues, slow the process of fibrosis.

Lumican

Lumican can be found in organs as well as the eye. It combines with keratin sulfate in the eye to create a transparent cornea. Too many glycosaminoglycans attached to lumican in an organ such as the heart are seen after injury as part of the remodeling of that tissue. Too much lumican in the kidney can exacerbate chronic kidney disease.

Fibromodulin

Fibromodulin is a regulator of lysyl oxidase, the enzyme which cross-links collagen. Fibromodulin's presence may limit excessive cross-linking. It also binds growth factors and cytokines, with an overall anti-inflammatory and anti-angiogenic function.

Syndecan

Syndecan is a transmembrane protein that can bind to collagens, fibronectin, and growth factors. It has pro- and anti-inflammatory functions and can help white blood cells move along epithelial surfaces.

Proteins

There are roughly 300 proteins in the ECM. There are also many enzymes and growth factors nested in these structures. Collagen and elastin are key. In general, during hypofunction, the proteins of the ECM become deficient and develop excessive cross-linking in the case of collagen. Aging is a good example of hypofunction.

Collagen

There are at least 28 types of collagen in the ECM, with the fibril collagen types I, II, and III being the most common. Others such as V, VI, XIV, and XVII fibrillar collagens have interruptions in their triple helical structure. These are the backbone of the ECM and in fact the body, with approximately 30% of the body's protein being collagen, much of it fibrillar. Collagen is arrays in different directions in the ECM, which allows it to absorb stress coming from different directions. Fibrillar collagens are cross-linked by an enzyme called lysyl oxidase, weaving the helices of collagen into fibrils of varying thickness. Cross-linking provides more stability and eventually stiffness. Collagens IV, VIII, and X are used in the formation of mesh-like networks, with IV being predominant in basement membranes [1, 2].

Elastin

Elastin is a remarkable molecule that impacts stretch tolerance to tissues and has the property of returning energy to tissue. Elastic fibers are an elastin core surrounded by microfibrils. The latter are rich in fibrillin which is an extendible polymer that imparts many of the properties we associate with elastin. All tropoelastins share a characteristic domain arrangement of hydrophobic sequences alternating with lysine-containing cross-linking motifs. Microfibrillar proteins fibrillins and microfibril-associated glycoprotein-1 combine with elastin to make elastic fibers. There is a certain amount of cross-linking catalyzed by lysine oxidase (LOX enzymes, to bind elastic fibers together and to some collagen molecules. There are two major bifunctional cross-links in elastin: dehydrolysinonorleucine, formed through the condensation of one residue of allysine and one of lysine, and allysine aldol, formed through the association of two allysine residues. These two cross-links can further condense with each other, or with other intermediates, to form desmosine or isodesmosine. Cross-links impart strength to the elastin fibers.

Actin

Extracellular actin filaments are found throughout the ECM. These are used for cell motility. Cells can assemble and disassemble actin filaments that themselves are bound to proteins and this can create movement. These appendages that are created for this purpose are known as lamellipodia. Smaller actin filaments, called filopodia, can "reach out" from a cell to sense the environment.

Integrins

Integrins are the connection of the cell microtubules to the ECM. The ECM itself has connections to the cell via integrin molecules, which traverse the cell membrane. On the ECM side, the integrins connect with ECM proteins via fibronectin as a kind of coupling structure. Inside the cell, integrin is connected to the cytoskeleton via proteins such as talins and vinculins.

Integrins are produced by cells for their own cell membrane, and integrins can be released by fibroblasts, especially in the tumor microenvironment. In health, integrins are important for cellular migration, as they form a connection between cells and the actin filaments they might use to move. Integrins will bind to a fibronectin dimer, which creates a focal adhesion complex. The focal adhesion complex acts as a sensor of ECM laxity or stiffness and plays a major role in the mechanotransduction effects of the ECM on the cell and its nucleus (and mitochondria) [1, 2, 4, 5] (Fig. 2.1).

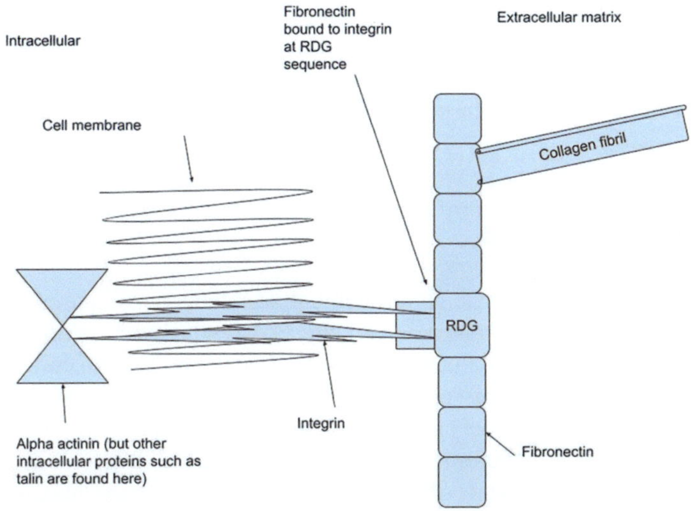

Fig. 2.1 Adhesion complex

Fibronectin

Fibronectin is a glycoprotein. This is similar to a proteoglycan, but a glycoprotein does not have repeating disaccharide units (but does have sugar and amine attachments in one molecule). It is usually in a dimeric form with a disulfide bond bridge. Fibronectin is important for connection of cells to the ECM and for cell migration.

Perlecan

Perlecan is a large membrane heparan sulfate proteoglycan. It is found in basement membranes, as well as very dense tissues such as cartilage. It assists in the polarization of epithelial cells at a basement membrane, helping them keep the apical (top) surface of the epithelium facing into the external environment or the lumen of an organ or duct. Its normal function is necessary for muscle and bone formation. Its dysfunction will allow cancer cells to invade their local environments and release angiogenic factors. Perlecans can bind to vegetative endothelial growth factors and fibroblast growth factors and initiate angiogenesis via Protein B (AKT) kinases and MAPK (mitogen-activated protein kinases).

Hyaluronic Acid

Hyaluronic acid is a glycosaminoglycan that is composed of repeating D-glucuronic acid and N-acetyl-D-glucosamine (disaccharides) joined by glucuronic bonds. There is no protein core to hyaluronic acid. It is extremely important for tissue hydration, and it forms a gel-like environment around cells. Cell migration is facilitated by hyaluronic acid. The brain has little structural protein but large amounts of hyaluronic acid. Skin has large amounts of it, as does cartilage. When it is broken down, as in injury, fragments of hyaluronic acid can bind to Toll-like receptors to activate inflammation. Although hyaluronic acid does not form covalent bonds with proteoglycans, it does aggregate with them using non-covalent attractions.

Laminin

Laminins are heterotrimeric (three stranded) glycoproteins that have a cross-like shape. They can bind to collagen type IV—mesh-forming fibrillar protein in basement membranes. Laminins (there are 15 members in this group) can influence cell adhesion, migration, and differentiation.

Nidogen-1

This protein used to be known as entactin. It interacts with Collagen IV and fibronectin and is found in basement membranes. It also interacts with cells and assists with the structural integrity of tissues and cell differentiation.

Tenascin

Tenascin has four subtypes and binds to collagen, fibronectin, proteoglycans, and growth factors. It is very involved in embryogenesis. It also has a role in cellular and tissue repair, as well as cell migration. When tissues are damaged, tenascin-C and other members of this group can become strong activators of the pattern recognition receptors such as Toll-like receptors. Tenascins act as DAMPs (damage-associated molecular patterns) that can provoke innate immune responses and inflammation.

Resident Cells

The proteins and proteoglycans of the ECM are extremely important, but the ECM has specialized cell populations. These cells deposit and maintain the matrix.

Fibroblasts

Fibroblasts are spindle-shaped cells that vary widely in their specific morphology, depending on the organ or tissue of residence. They can create strong and elastic lung ECM and resilient skin or muscle ECM. The heart has its own type of fibroblasts derived from progenitors (mostly from epicardium—the outer layer of the heart and some being endocardial). Fibroblasts are replicated with stimulation from platelet-derived growth factor.

They are the primary producers of the "matrisome"—the proteins of the ECM. This includes proteoglycans, collagen, elastin, and fibronectin. Fibroblasts also produce the enzymes that are essential for the maintenance of the matrix. These include matrix metalloproteinases (MMPs), which break down ECM proteins. Fibroblasts also secrete lysyl oxidases, which cross-link collagens in the ECM, giving stability and a certain degree of stiffness. Another product are the inhibitors of the MMP, specifically the tissue inhibitor of metalloproteinases (TIMP) which keep MMP activity in check. Fibroblasts secrete growth factors and adipokines (which are also secreted by adipose cells). In addition to creating the cross-linked collagen that can create matrix structure, fibroblasts can pull on the matrix causing cellular responses.

Fibroblasts are resident to the ECM, and under the influence of cytokines such as transforming growth factor beta and tumor necrosis factor alpha, they can transform into myofibroblasts. These contractile fibroblasts, which are capable of migrating through the ECM, are highly secretory and are integral to wound healing. They can also overproduce matrix proteins, leading to matrix stiffness. As we shall see in subsequent chapters, fibroblasts can overactivate due to inflammation and oxidative stress, with fibrosis being a typical and predictable outcome of long-term tissue/organ inflammation and decline.

Macrophages

Macrophages were described by Elie Metchnikoff, a Russian zoologist in 1884. These protective cells exist in the bloodstream and in the extracellular matrix. They engulf pathogens and destroy them and, in the process, present antigen to the rest of the immune system. Since T cells must "read" antigen by it being bound to major histocompatibility complex (MHC), macrophages use this protein in both its forms. Macrophage cell membrane MHC1 can present antigen to cytotoxic T cells (CD8), and MHCII can present antigen to help T cells (CD4).

Macrophages play a distinct role in the ECM. They are the primary remodelers of matrix by secreting matrix metalloproteinases. They also secrete multiple cytokines. Macrophages are now understood to be plastic and to polarize into either of two primary forms (which of course, may have subtypes). The classically activated or M1 macrophages are more defensive and can more powerfully upregulate inflammation. They are stimulated by pathogen-associated molecular patterns and Interferon gamma. The M1 secrete primarily: TNFα, IL-1, IL-6, IL-12, and IL-23 [1, 2].

Polarization to nonclassical M2 macrophages has several variants. The M2a type is created by IL-4 and IL-13 stimulation, and once so polarized, they secrete IL-10. The presence of IL-10 has a downregulating effect on inflammation.

Lipopolysaccharides (LPS), from the cell walls of gram-negative bacteria, along with IgG-immune complexes, can create M2b-type macrophages, which themselves secrete IL-10 which is auto-stimulatory. This is protective mechanism, as LPS is massively pro-inflammatory (activating pattern recognition receptors) and the ability of M2b and IL10 to quell that response prevents septic shock like conditions (to a point) [1, 2, 6].

IL-10, TGF-β, or glucocorticoids can create M2c macrophages, which are also matrix forming and can become pro-fibrotic. M2 macrophages also can secrete proteases, specifically MMP9, and this has a role in angiogenesis. The matrix disassembly due to MMP9 release makes room for the sprouting of new blood vessels.

In addition to MHC and T cell interactions, the role of macrophages in innate immune responses needs to be mentioned. Macrophages have Toll-like receptors on their surface and in their cytoplasm. They also have inflammasomes, which are intracellular processing bodies for antigen (which is ideal given the phagocytotic nature of the macrophage). This means that macrophages are powerful upregulatory of inflammation due to the recognition of damage associated with molecular patterns (fragments of nuclei, mitochondria, and extracellular matrix resulting from necrosis). Macrophages also react strongly to pathogen-associated molecular patterns as noted above. In a later chapter, we shall discuss the cancer-associated fibroblast, which retains the abilities of its original form but veers into a service role for neoplastic cells.

Tissue Specificity of ECM

Extracellular matrix is reflective of, and determinant of, the tissue type where it can be found [7, 8]. Cardiac ECM, for example, contains a lot of glycosaminoglycans including hyaluronan and heparin. The brain is very high in hyaluronic acid but very low in fibrous proteins. Bone contains much type 1 collagen and is structured to accept mineral crystals (hydroxyapatite). Lung tissue has plenty of collagen I and collagen type IV and fibronectin (as part of basement membranes) but also a great deal of elastin to allow it to resist stress and to have elastic recoil. Muscle extracellular matrix has distinct layers: epimysium, perimysium, and endomysium, which assist in the diffusion of calcium and contraction. Cartilage has very dense collagen type II and is glycosaminoglycans, as well as aggrecan to tie structures together tightly so that this structure can resist compression. Tendon ECM is extremely high in collagen, which is aligned along the long axis (directions of force) of the tendon, along with decorin, an SLRP. In the kidney, collagen IV, nidogen, and laminin are common features across the mesangial matrix, glomerular basement membrane, and Bowman's capsule, but there are differences, with the glomerular basement membrane having other collagen types plus the SLRP perlecan. Liver ECM has abundant type I and III collagen. Splenic ECM has many basement membrane-oriented components much like the kidney and also has collagen types I, II, and III, fibronectin, and tenascin-C.

Cellular Receptors That Interact with ECM

Cellular receptors for the ECM are explored in the upcoming chapter on physiology of the ECM. In general, the aforementioned integrins are important to connections of intracellular structures to the ECM and general force sensing of the cell. CD44 is a cell surface protein needed for adhesion, including attachment to actin and collagen. Discoidin domain receptors attach to collagen and, like integrin, can have second messenger systems set up on the intracellular side.

ECM Determinant Cell Differentiation and Behavior

The incredibly specialized and tissue-specific components of the ECM, and the specialized cells that inhabit it, are integral to cellular function. Although the cell as a unit can be studied in various models and mediums, in vivo, cells are truly inseparable from their extracellular matrix. This is more than just a proximity or physical hard connection—the function of cells and their phenotypic type are highly conditioned by the matrix.

References

1. Yue B. Biology of the extracellular matrix. J Glaucoma. 2014;23(8):S20–3.
2. Karamanos NK, Theocharis AD, Piperigkou Z, Manou D, Passi A, Skandalis SS, et al. A guide to the composition and functions of the extracellular matrix. FEBS J. 2021;288(24):6850.
3. Iozzo RV, Schaefer L. Proteoglycan form and function: a comprehensive nomenclature of proteoglycans. Matrix Biol. 2015;42(March):11–55.
4. Dalton CJ, Lemmon CA. Fibronectin: molecular structure, fibrillar structure and mechanochemical signaling. Cells. 2021;10(9):2443.
5. Berdiaki A, Neagu M, Tzanakakis P, Spyridaki I, Pérez S, Nikitovic D. Extracellular matrix components and mechanosensing pathways in health and disease. Biomol Ther. 2024;14(9):1186.
6. Meza-Morales W, Jimenez-Socha M, Freytes DO, Mora C. Macrophages and the extracellular matrix. In: Results and problems in cell differentiation; 2024. p. 55–87.
7. Mouw JK, Ou G, Weaver VM. Extracellular matrix assembly: a multiscale deconstruction. Nat Rev Mol Cell Biol. 2014;15(12):771–85.
8. McKee TJ, Perlman G, Morris M, Komarova SV. Extracellular matrix composition of connective tissues: a systematic review and meta-analysis. Sci Rep. 2019;9(1):10542.

Physiology of the Extracellular Matrix

3

The extracellular matrix (ECM) serves as support and structure for the body and has important functional roles. These physiological roles are often rooted in structures and connections of the ECM, cells, and their organelles [1–3].

Stability

The cell membranes have receptors such as integrins, discoidin domain receptors (DDRs), syndecans, and CD44. The anchors can attach to the ECM and somewhat fix the cell in place. This is important for epithelial cells in particular and helps them organization and polarity. Cells can be immobilized and anchored to the matrix and reciprocally help organize the ECM (Fig. 3.1). Without this stability, stem cells in adults cannot divide and differentiate (commit to a certain tissue type) properly.

Arginylglycylaspartic acid is also known as Arg-Gly-Asp (RGD). It acts as an adhesive, connecting the proteoglycans fibronectin, vitronectin, and tenascin to the cell. It binds directly to integrins, including $\alpha v\beta 3$ integrin [1].

Anokis is the term referring to the death of cells when they are detached from the extracellular matrix (Fig. 3.2). An intrinsic and extrinsic pathway that leads to a death program is ready to be activated in cells but is paused by attachments of focal adhesion com-

F. Smith, *The Extracellular Matrix in Health and Disease*,
https://doi.org/10.1007/978-3-031-94465-9_3

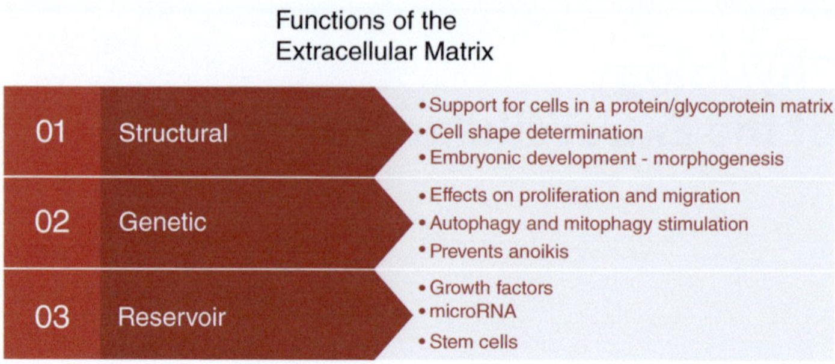

Fig. 3.1 Functions of the ECM

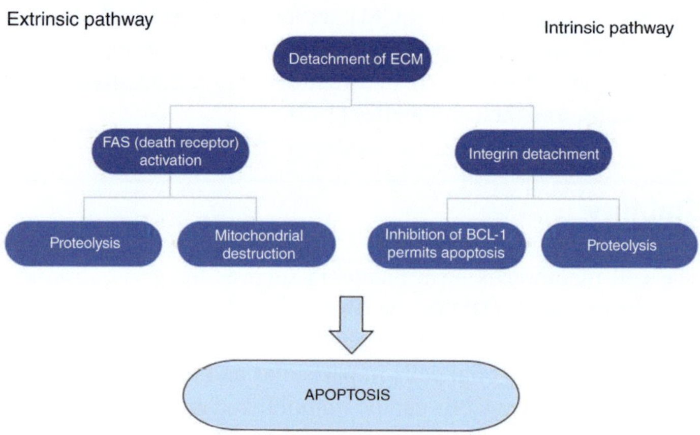

Fig. 3.2 Anoikis

plexes. If these are removed, the cell dies. This prevents cells from wandering and taking root in tissues where they do not belong. Cancer cells, unsurprisingly, can shut down the cell death program, detach themselves from the ECM, and go where they please [4].

Force Sensing and Mechanotransduction

The cell can sense ECM forces. This is due to binding of ECM structures to integrin on the cell surface (via fibronectin). On the cytoplasmic side, the cell has microtubules and microfilaments.

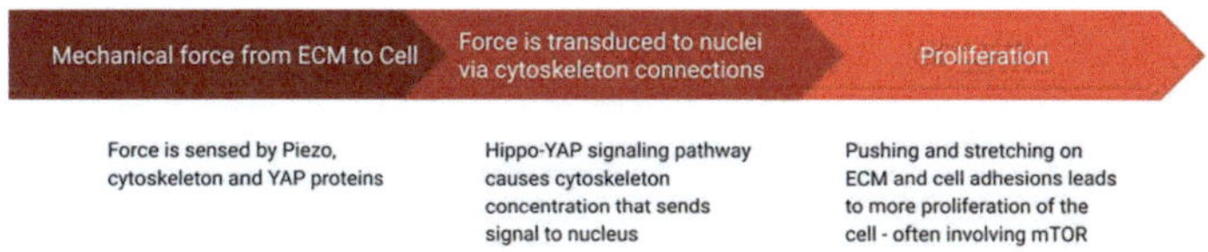

Fig. 3.3 Force sensing in ECM

These are bound to integrins, and also to organelles such as mitochondria, and to the nucleus. The stiffness of the matrix is transduced into a particular signal just as the softness of a matrix is. That has effects on cell division and migration (Fig. 3.3). It can also influence autophagy, the process by which damaged cellular proteins (including mitochondrial contents) are degraded to make room for new ones [5–7].

Cells experience push and pull phenomenon with the matrix and with other cells. The changes in orientation of cells and the density, alignment, and topography of ECM mean that a cell's behavior impacts its neighbors as well as the surrounding matrix. By the same token, forces sent via the matrix will reach the cell nucleus.

Intracellular signals also result from these forces, and the chemical signals that result from second messenger system, initiated by mechanical forces, are the true mechanotransduction.

Tana Rozario and Douglas W DeSimone (who was one of the first scientists to renew interest in and bring modern molecular biology to bear on the ECM) have characterized this touch, tug, pull, and mechanical transduction phenomena as a "morphogenetic language or code," one "that is interpreted by the cells that come in contact with it" [1].

Growth Factors

The ECM can bind and release growth factors such as vegetative endothelial growth factor and the concentration gradient for many growth factors, including bone morphogenetic proteins, the latter being part of the transforming growth factor (TGF)-type signaling molecule. TGF is in an inactive form in the ECM until proteases (such as MMP9), tenascin glycopro-

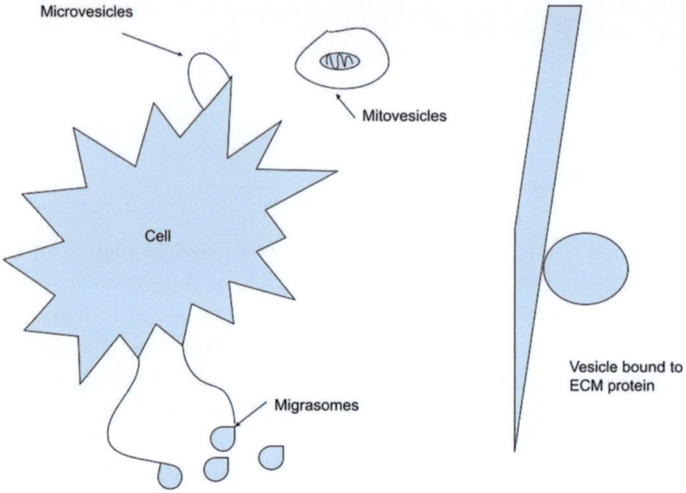

Fig. 3.4 Vesicles in ECM

teins (which have a domain that is very similar to TGF), or even changes in pH convert TGF into an active form. The ECM can be a reservoir for growth factors partly due to the charge of sulfated glycosaminoglycans, which attracts many growth factors. They can also be contained in vesicles, which are bound to proteoglycans, particularly small leucine rich proteoglycans. In addition to MMPs, other proteases such as ADAM (which stands for a disintegrin and metalloproteinase) play a major role in liberation of growth factors from matrix [8–10].

Other vesicles found in the ECM include migrasomes, which are outcroppings of cells in motion, containing mRNA [11]. And mitosomes are vesicles with mitochondrial components. Much is still being discovered about vesicles, but it is clear that they are important for cell-to-cell communication [12]. As is often the case, the extracellular matrix is the conduit of this communication (Fig. 3.4).

Proliferation

Cell proliferation is heavily influenced by the surrounding ECM. The ECM and its adhesions to the cell are needed for normal proliferation. An ECM that becomes stiffer enhances these adhesions and activates intracellular enzymes such as MAPK and Rho, with more proliferation.

As will be discussed in future chapters, too much ECM rigidity can induce hyperproliferation in neoplasia [8].

Migration

When nearby ECM is rearranged by metalloprotein actions, cells may be inclined to migrate into more porous areas of the surrounding matrix. Cells can move along matrix grooves or tunnels by the interaction with focal adhesion complexes with nearby proteins. Intracellular actin filaments can be bundled into groups of about 10–30 filaments, cross-linked by alpha-actinin. Myosin filaments can move across the action, using ATP (must like muscle contraction), to pull on the focal adhesion complexes. These complexes are, extracellularly, bound to fibronectin, which is bound to various ECM components. This is one way that cells can move through the ECM [1].

Stem Cell Niche

Stem cells are essential progenitor-reserved cells. They are of course extremely active during human embryonic development, which involves intensive ECM interaction [13]. That phase of life is outside of the scope of this book, but it is important to note that in adults. The ECM plays a major role in the availability of stem cells. The mechanotransduction effects, transmitted by focal adhesion complexes in stem cells, can increase activity (Fig. 3.5). A

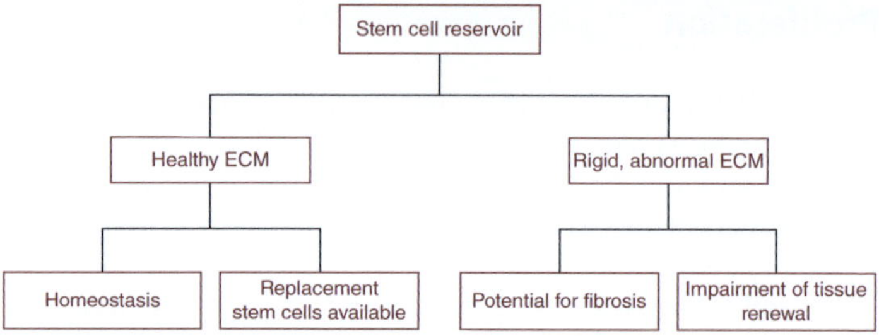

Fig. 3.5 Stem cell niche

matrix that is stiffer, which requires higher forces to strain and deform it, actually decreases stem cell activation. This is one problem facing aged ECM, but also diseased ECM, which can also sideline much needed, but unfortunately quiescent stem cells [1].

Neoplasia Resistance or Encouragement

A diseased ECM is often a welcoming environment for neoplastic cells. It is well established that cancer cells cultivate a specific ECM environment to help them survive, proliferate, and disseminate. It is also becoming clearer that some ECM types give the types of mechanotransduction signals to cells that encourage oncogenes to become more active. This is not surprising since the cell behavior and even differentiation follow matrix cues. This does not negate the importance of mutagenic and promotional events in the cancer development process. However the inflammatory, rigid, and overly stimulatory nature of some diseased matrices can encourage a cell in its anaplastic, dysplastic, and finally neoplastic journey [14].

Clinical Implications

A dysfunctional ECM is likely to foster dysfunction and progressive disease in the local tissue. Any diseased organ or tissue will have pathological changes to the ECM. Although cellular pathology remains a critical focal point of diagnosis, ECM is inextricably connected to the cell and so they share the responsibility for homeostasis and they both exhibit disease states.

Summary

The extracellular matrix is extremely active. Half a century of continuous and brilliant research into this substrate of cells has put to rest any archaic notions of the ECM as a mere "bulletin board" or cells. On the contrary, the ECM is active and interactive with cells. It is influenced by cell behavior, but itself is a determinant of cell fate. The concept of "dynamic interplay" is applied to this relationship. Cells are not really independent of an ECM, although they can be studied apart from it to gain knowledge. In living organisms, cells and surrounding ECM practically form a life unit. Since many determinants of health and disease happen within the ECM and the ECM cell interface, this is a critical area to explore the ways in which naturopathic medicine approaches can be effective. The subsequent chapters of this book discuss that very question. This is proffered with the humility that this discussion is simply one small slice of the vast trove of ECM research and only one dimension of what naturopathic treatment can be.

References

1. Rozario T, DeSimone DW. The extracellular matrix in development and morphogenesis: a dynamic view. Dev Biol. 2010;341(1):126–40.
2. Klein EA, Castagnino P, Kothapalli D, Yin L, Byfield FJ, Xu T, et al. Cell cycle control by physiological matrix elasticity and in vivo tissue stiffening. Curr Biol. 2009;19(18):1511–8.
3. Muncie JM, Weaver VM. The physical and biochemical properties of the extracellular matrix regulate cell fate. Curr Top Dev Biol. 2018;130:1–37.
4. Taddei M, Giannoni E, Fiaschi T, Chiarugi P. Anoikis: an emerging hallmark in health and diseases. J Pathol. 2011;226(2):380–93.
5. Plotnikov Sergey V, Pasapera Ana M, Sabass B, Waterman CM. Force fluctuations within focal adhesions mediate ECM-rigidity sensing to guide directed cell migration. Cell. 2012;151(7):1513–27.

6. Humphrey JD, Dufresne ER, Schwartz MA. Mechanotransduction and extracellular matrix homeostasis. Nat Rev Mol Cell Biol. 2014;15(12):802–12.
7. Berdiaki A, Neagu M, Tzanakakis P, Spyridaki I, Pérez S, Nikitovic D. Extracellular matrix components and mechanosensing pathways in health and disease. Biomol Ther. 2024;14(9):1186.
8. Lu P, Takai K, Weaver VM, Werb Z. Extracellular matrix degradation and remodeling in development and disease. Cold Spring Harb Perspect Biol. 2011;3(12):a005058.
9. Bonnans C, Chou J, Werb Z. Remodelling the extracellular matrix in development and disease. Nat Rev Mol Cell Biol. 2014;15(12):786–801.
10. Al Halawani A, Mithieux SM, Yeo GC, Hosseini-Beheshti E, Weiss AS. Extracellular vesicles: interplay with the extracellular matrix and modulated cell responses. Int J Mol Sci. 2022;23(6):3389.
11. Zhang X, Yao L, Meng Y, Li B, Yang Y, Gao F. Migrasome: a new functional extracellular vesicle. Cell Death Discov. 2023;9(1):381.
12. D'Acunzo P, Kim Y, Ungania JM, Pérez-González R, Goulbourne CN, Levy E. Isolation of mitochondria-derived mitovesicles and subpopulations of microvesicles and exosomes from brain tissues. Nat Protoc. 2022;17(11):2517–49.
13. Linde-Medina M, Marcucio R. Living tissues are more than cell clusters: the extracellular matrix as a driving force in morphogenesis. Prog Biophys Mol Biol. 2018;137:46–51.
14. Cox TR. The matrix in cancer. Nat Rev Cancer. 2021;21(4)

Levels of Dysfunction and Impact on and of the Extracellular Matrix

4

In this book, a model of the levels of dysfunction is used [1]. This model traces the progression of dysfunction in an organ or tissue from superficial and transient to substantial and irreversible. By dysfunction, we mean a decline in the ability of that organ or tissue's ability to function and perform its normal role. The mildest and most easily correctable level of dysfunction is that of simply hypofunction. This is when an organ or tissue is intact structurally but performs at a less than optimal level. This is not commensurate with actual pathology, and it may produce actual symptoms but they may be subtle. Or they may be general in nature, such as fatigue. Hypofunction commonly emerges when some determining factors of health are not adequately met. For example, in dehydration, the mucosa of the bronchial passages becomes more congested as the mucus becomes more viscous. This is not a cause of actual asthma, but it will exacerbate it and, under certain conditions, might be noticeable to a non-asthmatic (such as during more intense bouts of exercise). Another kind of hypofunction might be a slight reduction in the production of thyroid hormone. This might not be to the level of clinical hypothyroidism, but the person may notice a reduction in energy to complete tasks and a tendency to put on weight (Fig. 4.1).

The next level of dysfunction is that of impaired circulation and communication. This is an extension of hypofunction but with more noticeable obstruction and failure to coordinate organ

F. Smith, *The Extracellular Matrix in Health and Disease*,
https://doi.org/10.1007/978-3-031-94465-9_4

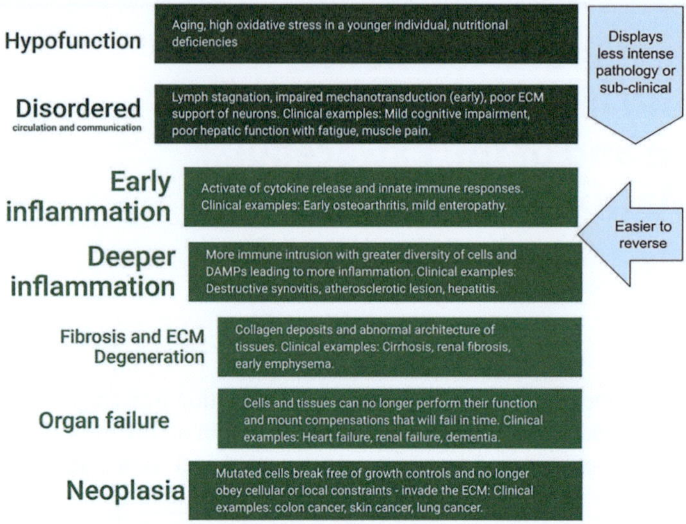

Fig. 4.1 Levels of dysfunction

functions. This stage is very likely to produce noticeable symptoms and signs. The patient will notice limitations of function more frequently and perhaps have complaints that they wish to discuss with a doctor. It is possible to live with a certain amount of impaired circulation and communication in a local tissue, although increasing reliance on symptom-suppressing treatments and avoidance of certain activities is likely. An example of this level would be a reduction in microcirculation in a muscle, including the heart. This can happen because of inflammation that somewhat occludes the microvasculature in some areas or simple recession of microvascular beds due to prolonged sedentary ways. The muscle or tissue in question is not in a state of acute ischemic stress and necrosis but will begin to atrophy and will not perform within a normal physiological range. A patient with impaired coronary microvascular function will be fatigued and may have heart failure (early) type signs, even though the major coronary arteries are still reasonably patent. Or, a decrease in nerve conduction velocity due to glycation damage in diabetes mellitus leads to poor sensory inputs and decreased motor coordination (a phenomenon that involves local nerves, the spinal cord pathways, and the brain). The blockages and discord that occur in this level of dysfunction will tend to cause progressive symptoms and, in many cases, inflammation. For example, as microcirculation becomes progressively impaired, minute ischemic events can lead to localized reperfusion injuries—tolerable at first, but the cumulative effect of these insults will eventually cause inflammation and disease.

Initial inflammation is the next level of dysfunction. This can be a helpful response, and it is a predictable and necessary response to injury. The remodeling that occurs during the resolution of inflammation can lead to actual healing. However, an overly robust inflammatory response can be destructive. Some inflammatory events can become medical emergencies. More commonly, inflammation is chronic and, in time, will shift to a higher intensity type. An example would be osteoarthritis where some inflammatory damage is occurring, even though it is not an inflammatory or autoimmune type of arthritides. Dietary factors and other disturbances to the determining factors of health can make these joints more painful. Or, earlier stage cardiovascular disease is characterized by upticks in inflammatory biomarkers, and oxidation of low density lipoprotein (LDL) particles (the APO-A subunit of) even before atheromatous plaques is well established. Inflammation is a protective response that allows innate and more selective immune forces to enter a region of the body. It is an attempt to rectify a disturbance or obstruction. But if the causative effects of inflammation are not removed, then it becomes chronic, and this is usually progressive in nature.

Deeper inflammation is characterized by the loss of downregulating factors that would squelch inflammation and move a tissue to a resolution and healing phase. There are many causes of chronic inflammation including ongoing disturbances to the determining factors of health, recurring infections, and autoimmune reactions to body tissues. Moreover, the damage-associated molecular patterns (DAMPs) created by the destruction of cells bind to sensors of cell and tissue damage (pattern recognition receptors or PRRs). That binding to PRR, such as Toll-like receptors, activates inflammation, which can damage cells and extracellular matrix, thereby creating more DAMPs, and so on. Although the body can tolerate ongoing inflammation for a while, eventually it leads to an increasingly maladaptive state.

The extracellular matrix in inflammation shows all of the classic responses to injury features. Macrophages can polarize to M1 early in the inflammation and behave destructively but then polarize to M2 during resolution. Matrix metalloproteinases, essential for normal maintenance of the ECM, as well as ADAM enzymes, become overproduced, which leads to destruction of the ECM. The various glycoproteins of the ECM can become damaged, and the collagens cross-linked to the point that they lose they start providing maladaptive signaling to the cells.

The next step in ongoing inflammation, persistent failure of circulation of nutrients and communication between cells, and progressive damage is a predictable response for any tissue that has been repeatedly damaged. This involves fibrosis of some kind, the elaboration of scar tissue that results from overactivation of fibroblasts when a tissue has repeatedly been injured. This almost always involves transformation of fibroblasts to myofibroblasts, which secrete collagen exuberantly. For example, the liver will elaborate fibrous tissue after repeated insults, to the point that cirrhosis of the liver can make the organ nonviable.

The elaboration of fibrotic tissue in fact cross cuts the vital extracellular matrix. The ECM, the central topic of this book, is essential for cell maintenance, nourishment, toxin disposal, growth signaling, gene transcription, immune activation, and more. When the ECM itself begins to crumble, or stiffens up to the point where it becomes nonelastic and nonporous, and has an abnormal topography, the very tissue and its cells are destined to die. This is the gateway to organ failure.

In organ failure, the ECM no longer has the architectural features to support cellular life. For example, in the kidney, ECM degradation leads to loss of filtration actions. In the heart, the ECM dissolution leads to loss of support for action/myosin-containing cardiomyocytes. In the brain, "failure" is too generalized a word, but in some areas, an abnormal matrix will inhibit myelination, and in others, it can cause more inflammation and more neuron destruction.

Neoplasia will get special consideration in this book. A surprising amount of events occur in the ECM in neoplastic events. The term "tumor microenvironment" encompasses this. Cancer cells not only exploit damaged ECM. The neoplastic cells actively sculpt the ECM to serve its own goals of immune evasion, uncontrolled growth, seizure of nutrients from the rest of the body, and of course local and distal spread. This is all brokered by the ECM.

In the chapters that follow, we will examine these levels of dysfunction and how they impact the extracellular matrix. The role of naturopathic therapies to offset these problems is addressed, with specific recommendations. It should be noted that the examples provided, while relevant, are only a cross section of the many types of treatments in naturopathic medicine. The direct effects of these treatments in any specific patient situation are not always measurable, at least in a practice versus a research context. Nevertheless, the purpose of naturopathic medicine is to create the conditions for health and to remove the obstacles to healing. Taking specific actions to protect and rehabilitate the extracellular matrix is very much in line with the principles and practices of naturopathic medicine.

Diagnosis

The research methodologies in exploring the ECM in disease have advanced rapidly in the past three decades. These methods have not reached the bedside yet, but in time, they could become powerful modes of insight into health and disease.

Some examples of ECM analysis are explained in the excellent 2023 review by Park et al.

Strategic outline of interventions targeting extracellular matrix for promoting healthy longevity [2].

These include the matreotype [2, 3], which uses mass spectrometry or immunohistochemistry to identify the particular composition of matrix proteins in a sample. This can compare tissue-specific samples to their more typical configuration. This creates a type of "fingerprint" [2] of the matrix proteins.

Even blood samples can reveal telltale collagen fragments that are products of matrix metalloproteinase actions, which might be present in unusual levels. Specific molecules can also be extracted from a sample of tissue using magnetic nano-tweezers [4].

For the time being, clinicians will need to fall back on the more carefully studied and known changes to ECM that accompany various disease states. But the promise of the future is the development of direct diagnostic methods, as these migrate, in some form, from lab bench to bedside.

Level of dysfunction	Hallmarks	Changes in the ECM
Hypofunction	Decreased function and signs of change away from normal, but few visible signs or pronounced symptoms	Increase in cross-linked collagen but not to the point of fibrosis; persistence of senescent fibroblasts
Disordered communication and circulation	Blood, lymph, and nervous system flow or coordination are either impaired or dysregulated	Lymph exchange in proximity to the ECM is reduced; nutrients and signaling compounds to and from the cell are less available; changes to ECM begin to impact cellular function
Early inflammation	Innate immune responses are activated; macrophages enter M1 polarity	Some disruption due to matrix metalloproteinase and ADAM enzymes; chemoattraction of neutrophils and lymphocytes
Deeper inflammation	A wider array of immune components become involved and tissue destruction becomes more prominent—the risks of self-perpetuating inflammation increase	More extensive dissolution of structures; release of pro-inflammatory cytokines; increased expression of CD44 and more white blood cell intrusion into the ECM; cellular necrosis and ECM degradation create damage-associated molecular patterns that activate more inflammation via pattern recognition receptors; more immune cells engage with the tissue

Level of dysfunction	Hallmarks	Changes in the ECM
Fibrosis and extracellular matrix degeneration	As a reaction to significant damage, various myofibroblasts (depending on tissue—can be glial and astrocyte cells in brain) elaborate excessive collagen	The ECM can become filled with cross-linked collagen and a pathological increase in stiffness that impacts cellular phenotypes, cell division, mitochondrial function, etc. The original architecture of the ECM is now altered, often permanently Lack of autophagy and induction of a senescent phenotype begin
Organ failure	Change to the structure of the organ and loss of viable cells impair the basic functions of the organ; fundamental homeostats are not operating; allostasis and then heterostasis set in, until these compensations fail	The ECM, because of fundamental alterations to its architecture and composition, can do longer support the essential functions of the cells and the tissues. Impaired autophagy and a pro-senescent phenotype are worsened by damaged ECM and will in turn damage organs even further
Neoplasia	A colony of mutated cells break free from local controls and begin a program of invasion, at the expense of the host	A sequence of movements into the ECM are typical of many tumors—increased inflammation with the appearance of desmoplasia around the tumor, followed by excessive degradation of the ECM in order to release growth/angiogenic factors from their binding sites in the ECM and to spread cancer cells

Adapted from Smith [1]

References

1. Smith F. Naturopathic medicine. Cham: Springer; 2022.
2. Park JYC, King A, Björk V, English BW, Fedintsev A, Ewald CY. Strategic outline of interventions targeting extracellular matrix for promoting healthy longevity. Am J Physiol Cell Physiol. 2023;325(1):C90–128.
3. Ewald C. The matrisome during aging and longevity: a systems-level approach toward defining matreotypes promoting healthy aging. Gerontology. 2019;66(3):1–9.
4. Aermes C, Hayn A, Fischer T, Mierke CT. Environmentally controlled magnetic nano-tweezer for living cells and extracellular matrices. Sci Rep. 2020;10(1):13453.

5 Naturopathic Therapeutics and Effects on the Extracellular Matrix

The extracellular matrix is a pervasive network which spans the human organism, giving support to cells and exerting profound influences on their activity. This connection spans the nuclear matrix to cytoplasm, to integrin, to the extracellular matrix proteins and glycoproteins, linking the entire organism together. Cells interact with the matrix via cell surface receptors including CD44 (hyaluronan and others), discoidin domain receptors (collagens), cell surface proteoglycans (fibronectin and others), and integrins (major extracellular matrix [ECM] ligands including, fibronectin, vitronectin, fibrinogen, collagens, and laminins) [1].

One immediate conclusion about this totality of connections is that stimuli, or trauma, to one area is likely to be "perceived" in others. The nature of the communication across the ECM is still being understood, but mechanotransduction appears to be an important aspect of it [2].

Another conclusion is that therapies that influence or stimulate the ECM can cause whole system impacts. These could include manual medicine, acupuncture, electrical therapies, hydrotherapy, the old nature cure modalities of air and sun baths, homeopathy, and more. This is in essence the leveraging of the physical, hard-wired nature of the ECM to cell membrane to nucleus axis. This has been referred to as morphogenic inputs and is a powerful and primitive form of communication across living organisms [3].

F. Smith, *The Extracellular Matrix in Health and Disease*,
https://doi.org/10.1007/978-3-031-94465-9_5

Finally, the molecular biology of the ECM is amenable to influences by plant extracts, and nutrients, and the purposeful use of these therapies can protect, regenerate, regulate, and repair the ECM. It is important to realize that the ECM is yet another complex system in the body (joined by others such as nervous, endocrine, and immune) that responds to inputs from physicians but is not completely governed by them. It is self-regulating. This also means that plant extracts and nutrients that have one effect on one type of ECM, such as that ECM which has changed structurally after trauma, will not necessarily have an identical effect on ECM which is changing due to inflammation, breakdown, or even neoplasia.

Network Effects of Therapies on ECM

Acupuncture meridians are an integral concept in Traditional Chinese Medicine and similar systems. Acupuncture points are specific areas accessible from the skin where acupuncture needles are inserted (or pressure applied in some therapies). This system of treatment is centuries old with evidence of usage going back a couple of millennia. The acupuncture points are organized in sequences that run from distal fingers to the head or chest or distal toes to the head or chest. These are associated with specific organs. The insertion and manipulation of an acupuncture needle into a specific point on the meridian are done to influence the flow of body energies and fluids and the balance of Yin and Yang (fundamental energetic properties in that system) in a particular organ. Acupuncture is a widely used therapy across the world, with a great deal of documented and researched effects and benefits.

Insightful researchers have noticed that the route of acupuncture meridians is somewhat akin to that of various fascial tracks in the body. Investigations into this with human, animal, and dissection studies have found that acupuncture points enter into proximity with neurovascular bundles that are adjacent to fascial planes. The extensive networking of fibroblasts and their sensitivity to mechanotransduction provides a vehicle for activation via manual, acupuncture needle, laster, or microcurrent stimulation (Fig. 5.1). The many nerve endings and sensory receptors in the fascia and the ECM allow for further responsiveness to physical-therapeutic inputs [4, 5].

Neurovascular bundles are places where nerves and veins are fastened to connective tissue (Fig. 5.2). Fascia itself is connected to the extracellular matrix, with myofibroblasts that contribute the proteins of the fascia. Muscle fibers also digitate into the fascia. When an acupuncture needle is inserted into an acupuncture point, it is entering a particularly sensitive area of nerve, fascial, and extracellular matrix stimulation.

Electroacupuncture, where very small currents are fed into an inserted acupuncture needle, was found in a mouse model to create an antidepressant effect, possibly caused by increased matrix metalloproteinase expression, and an adaptive remodeling that can repair neural circuits and promote synaptic plasticity [6].

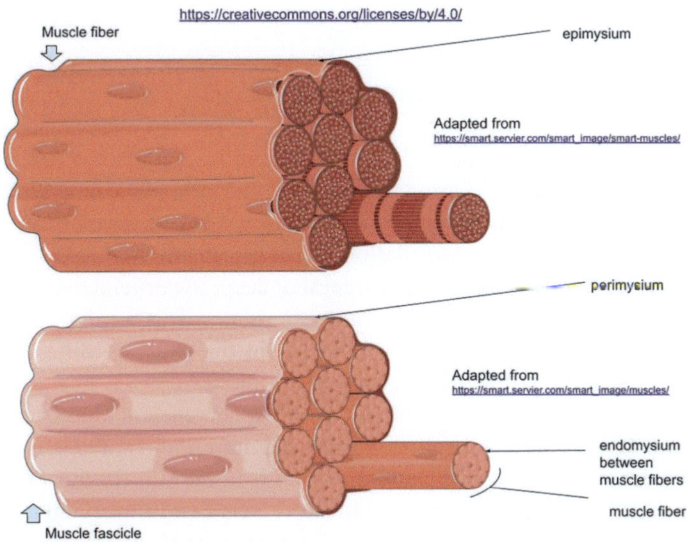

Fig. 5.1 Fascia and muscle

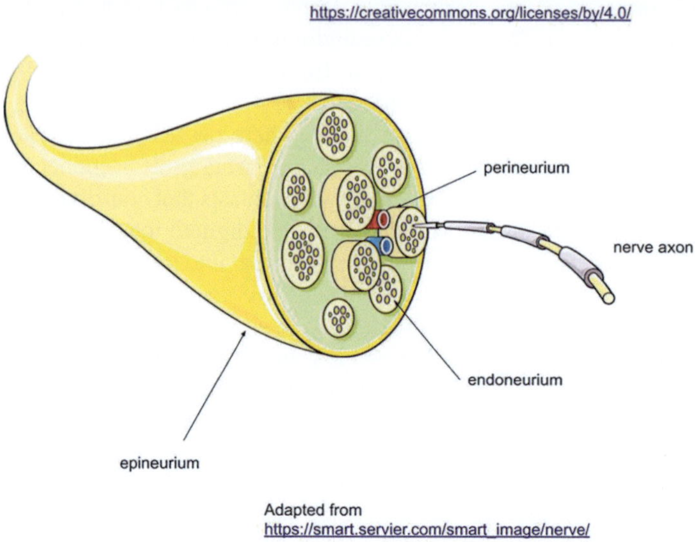

Fig. 5.2 Nerve ECM

Fascia as a Predominant Network

The fascial network pervades the body and is in contact with the extracellular matrix. Fascia is one of the first structures, emerging from the mesoderm layer divided during week 2 of development during the embryo's gastrulation phase [7]. It provides structure and support. Fascia can be superficial or deep. Superficial fascia is below the skin and superficial adipose tissues. It is a mixture of collagen and elastin fibers and varies in thickness in different regions. Muscle fibers sometimes insert into it.

Deep fascia surrounds bones, muscles, nerves, and blood vessels. It may have denser collagen and importantly and has a greater hyaluronic acid content, which is important for the sliding function that muscles need to have. Nerve endings, lymphatics, and a robust blood supply support this extensive network of deep fascia. Aponeurotic fascia can be fan shaped and act as an anchor a muscle to other muscular structures or even form tendons. The epimysial fascia wraps around muscle groups, and itself can connect to periosteal linings of bone. Large muscle groups naturally contain a lot of this kind of fascia, such as the gluteal muscles.

The fascia is embedded in extracellular matrix and is innervated [8]. Fibroblasts are predominant in fascia and can create the collagen structures of fascia and of the extracellular matrix. Fibroblasts act as a network through the fascial planes. In addition to well-known cytokine signaling that influences fibroblasts and the effects of matrix stiffness on fibroblasts, there are strong effects on fibroblasts via mechanotransduction [8]. This means that physical, including manual effects of stretch and compression, can activate the fibroblast network, which has therapeutic possibilities given the extent to which fibroblasts govern the ECM and the fascial structures.

Fasciacytes are cells along the margins of fascial structures that secrete hyaluronic acid, which helps with the sliding actions of fascia on other structures (including other fascia which is formed in layers). Fasciacytes are a fibroblast and can account for up to 30% of the fibroblast population in fascia [9].

Myofibroblasts have a contractile function and working in unison they can contract the extracellular matrix. A more recently discovered and yet to be fully understood cell is the telocytes. These have been identified as a network by Dawidowicz et al., and they possess extensions called telopods, which allow them to make local connections [10].

There are many nerve endings in the ECM and fascia, as well as numerous sensory receptors: muscle spindles (epimysial fasciae), the Golgi tendon organ, and Pacinian and Ruffini corpuscles (aponeurotic fasciae).

Effects of Nutrients on ECM Composition and Function

Although dietary components such as flavonoids have extensive effects on the ECM, the essential macro- and micronutrients also impact this system. Macronutrients are the lipids (fats), proteins (amino acids), and carbohydrates (complex and sugars). Micronutrients include the vitamins (fat and water soluble) and minerals (basic and trace). Since these nutrients are essential for normal structure and function, they are needed for the ECM. Protein is clearly essential for the ECM, since the amino acids from the diet are needed to make ECM proteins such as collagen and elastin. The ECM is also very rich in proteoglycans and glycoproteins which require amino acids. Enzymes such as matrix metalloproteinases are needed for remodeling of the ECM, and these are constructed out of amino acids. The proteins that connect the ECM, cells, and basement membranes in some cases, such as integrins, fibronectin, and laminin, as examples, are also dependent on adequate dietary protein [11].

As the name implies, glycoproteins and proteoglycans have sugar components, often repeating disaccharide units. Lipids are the basis of the cell and organelle membranes which the ECM connects with.

Vitamins and minerals in general are "required" for cellular metabolism and body function, but a few stand out in the ECM. Zinc is critical for protein synthesis, and, importantly, it is a catalyst for the aptly named matrix metalloproteinases [12].

Vitamin A is a widely deficient and integral to the ECM nutrient. It is required for production of collagen, laminin, entactin, fibronectin, elastin, and proteoglycans [13, 14]. Vitamin A deficiency is common worldwide, with the greatest prevalence in developing countries. US values for vitamin A are good, although people with malabsorption conditions can fail to reach their daily requirements. Likewise, those who assiduously avoid fat, who follow diet plans and fad erratically, or who eat excessive processed food can have values that are not a frank deficiency but are suboptimal. There are those who have mutations in the genes that produce the retinoid receptors in the cells, and like any polymorphism that impacts the role of a nutrient, their needs will be much greater for Vitamin A (Fig. 5.3).

Vitamin A deficiency leads to abnormal basement membrane formation, which has a serious impact on renal function. Collagen is produced in heaped up, irregular arrays, and lack of matrix

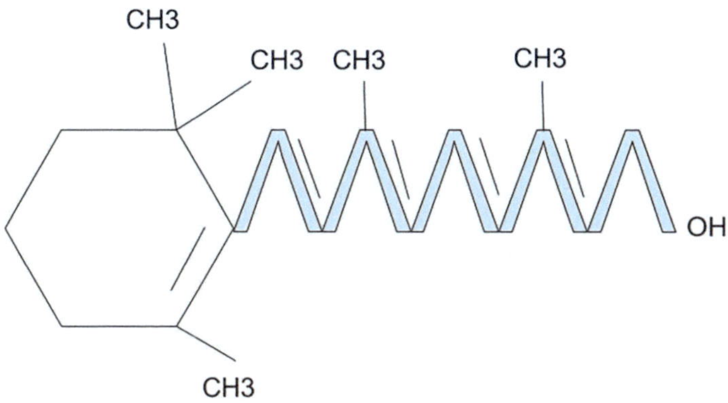

Fig. 5.3 Vitamin A

metalloproteinase function compounds the problem. This reduces the glomerular function.

In Vitamin A-deficient animals, the lung collagen, elastin, and laminin levels decrease. In the liver, vitamin A deficiency leads to overactivation of hepatic stellate cells, which lose their vitamin A content and transform into myofibroblasts which can proceed to secrete overabundant collagen. This can lead to fibrosis.

Vitamin D is another fat soluble vitamin that can be deficient. People in northern latitudes will automatically have limited sun exposure for a part of the year, and Vitamin D needs can increase for other reasons: diet, poor metabolic activation of vitamin D precursors, malabsorption, etc. [15] Although scientific debate is ongoing about the value of supplementation beyond an amount needed to sustain bone density, there is no doubt that many people across the world are deficient. Moreover, guidelines for D can be based on research on fairer skinned subjects who will produce more D in sunlight exposure than those with darker skin. If 800 IU of D is often enough to prevent deficiency in many, and 2000 IU per day should prevent deficiency in most adults, then clearly many people are not at adequate levels.

Vitamin D is required for extracellular matrix homeostasis [16]. It does so specifically by modulating the activity of matrix metalloproteinases which remodel and maintain the ECM. These include: Tissue inhibitor of metalloproteinases 1, 2, and 3 and matrix metalloproteinases 2 and 9.

Vitamin E, which has important roles as an antioxidant and cell and for organelle membrane stability, also reduces over activation of MMP by free radical scavenging. More directly, Vitamin E has some downregulating effect on MAPK (mitogen-activated protein kinase), which has effects on regulating MMP activity. Vitamin E is available in the germ of grains, eggs, nuts, seafood, and natural and unprocessed oils. It is a natural protector of lipids; hence it is found in undamaged fat contained foods. The proclivity for and abundance of ultra-processed foods in the diets of many leads to a reduction in available dietary E, along with an overabundance in polyunsaturated fatty acids, which by their nature require tocopherols for protection from oxidation.

Vitamin K, in terms of human requirements, is either K1 (phylloquinone) or K2 (menaquinones). Vitamin K1 is found in leafy green vegetables, such as kale or green leaf lettuce. Vitamin K2 is produced in the gut by the microbes there and then absorbed into the body. Some animal foods, such as liver, will have been synthesized by the human intestinal microbiota. A synthetic and not dietary form is K3 (menadione).

Vitamin K has well-known and essential functions in blood clotting and bone mineralization. It may also regulate MMP-2 and MMP-9, including that induced by the potent tissue plasminogen activator [17]. Although dietary intakes of K appear adequate for the majority of Americans, their actual K status might be impaired. The contribution of K from the gut may be less than anticipated, and the bioavailability of some dietary sources may be poor.

Folic acid is a required nutrient, needed for methylation processes throughout the body. There are dietary deficiencies, and there are polymorphisms that render people less able to efficiently activate the dietary folate into an active form using the enzyme methylenetetrahydrofolate reductase (MTHFR). This enzyme is needed for change of 5,10-methylene-tetrahydrofolate to 5-methylTHF. This leads to overactivation of MMP2 (via decrease methylation of the MM2 gene), damage to the decorin proteins in the ECM, and a more disorganized ECM [18]. Treatment with 5-methyltetrahydrofolate can bypass the relative deficiency in the

MTHFR activity. This is important for ECM integrity and may be of importance for those with various connective tissue issues and hypermobility syndromes.

Lymphatic Flow

The lymph system is critical for the drainage of fluid that runs from capillaries to lymphatic vessels [1]. This fluid has a draining and cleansing action on the extracellular matrix. Cells can discharge toxins into the ECM and thus into lymph. Tissues must expel wastes in this manner, and even the brain does this through the so-called "glymphatic" system. Lymph nodes, which are found along the course of this system, are loaded with antigen presenting dendritic cells and lymphocytes for the purpose of antigen recognition and immune response.

When the ECM is fibrotic, filled with cross-linked collagen, or extremely disorganized, lymph will have difficulty flowing through this area. Inflammation can contribute to this problem. Blocked lymphatics and localized lymphedema will in themselves lead to inflammation.

Treatment to increase the flow of lymph includes nutritional, physical-manual, and herbal therapies. Complete decongestive therapy is the standard medical approach. This involves manual therapy to increase lymph circulation, bandages, and physiological therapeutics. Manual therapies to increase lymph flow include drainage of individual limbs with specific strokes and overall body massage to move lymph back to the center of the body [19].

Botanical medicines can increase lymph flow. This has long been observed with herbs such as *Galium aparine* (Cleavers). Botanicals have compounds such as benzopyrones in the form of furanocoumarins, which help macrophages clear excessive fibrin and collagen deposition in the extracellular matrix. They may also help with activation of small blood vessels to help remove trapped fluid in an interstitial area. This is a feature of lymphedema as well as lipedema, which is a fluid infiltration and trapping in the ECM of adipose tissue. Flavonoids are also useful in lymph flow in the sense of improving the structural integrity of lymphatic vessels, and these are found in citrus fruits (hesperidin being one example) and berries such as *Vaccinium myrtillus* (bilberry). Saponins from the extract of *Aesculus hippocastanum* (Horse chestnut) and *Ruscus aculeatus* can somewhat vasoconstrict tiny blood vessels and prevent some fluid extravasation [20].

Exercise is valuable to move lymph, and exercise in the water, particularly slightly warm water, is used for people with lymphedema. Some patients report benefits from "rebounding"—using a small trampoline for daily exercise [21].

Botanical medicine directly impacting the extracellular matrix can take a number of pathways. Bioflavonoids, a broad category of molecules, have two phenolic rings and a carbon bridge. The types of flavonoids most likely to be found in foods (and supplements) include flavonols, flavan-3-ols, flavonols, flavanones, flavones, isoflavones, and anthocyanidins (which are more complex sheets of polyphenols).

These compounds have the ability to influence cell signaling pathways. They are also antioxidants, but their true value is most likely the influence on cellular behavior. Flavonoids can influence inflammasomes, mitogen-activated protein kinase, various matrix metalloproteinases, and even cytokines. These enzymes and signaling molecules are integral to the organization and function of the extracellular matrix.

The Importance of Generalized Treatment

We will discuss in this book ways in which common motifs play out in the ECM under different circumstances. Conditions that injure and degrade the ECM, such as oxidative stress, high serum glucose levels, and prolonged inflammation, lead to predictable outcomes. Reactions to these insults can repair the ECM but often do so in a form that is less than optimal. Sometimes, the repair process is so exuberant that the architecture of the regional ECM is alternated and assumes a less than functional state.

Some of the following chapters discuss the importance of dietary practices that provide nutrients that build and protect the ECM and that decrease inflammation in the body (or at least, the potential for excessive inflammation). A common problem today is the fact that many people enter a sentence association secretory phenotype, with extensive oxidative stress, glucose and insulin dysregulation, inflammation, and damage to ECM proteins. This causes organs to begin to dysfunction and inhibits the availability of much needed stem cells on the periphery of such tissues.

A useful model for examining what kind of measures can be taken to support the ECM, and health, can be found in the consideration of the level of dysfunction. This tells us something about the degree of disturbance and the kinds of events occurring in the matrix in question.

References

1. Wiig H, Keskin D, Kalluri R. Interaction between the extracellular matrix and lymphatics: consequences for lymphangiogenesis and lymphatic function. Matrix Biol. 2010;29(8):645–56.
2. Berdiaki A, Neagu M, Tzanakakis P, Spyridaki I, Pérez S, Nikitovic D. Extracellular matrix components and mechanosensing pathways in health and disease. Biomol Ther. 2024;14(9):1186.
3. Iozzo RV, Gubbiotti MA. Extracellular matrix: the driving force of mammalian diseases. Matrix Biol. 2018;71:1–9.
4. Maurer N, Nissel H, Egerbacher M, Gornik E, Schuller P, Traxler H. Anatomical evidence of acupuncture meridians in the human extracellular matrix: results from a macroscopic and microscopic interdisciplinary multicentre study on human corpses. Evid Based Complement Alternat Med. 2019;2019:1–8.
5. Bai Y, Wang J, Wu J, Dai J, Sha O, Tai Wai Yew D, et al. Review of evidence suggesting that the fascia network could be the anatomical basis for Acupoints and meridians in the human body. Evid Based Complement Alternat Med. 2011;2011:1–6.
6. Feng Y, Zhu G, Chen R, Shi G, Peng M, Zhou Y, et al. Electroacupuncture remodels the extracellular matrix and promotes synaptic plasticity in a mouse model of depression. Biochem Biophys Res Commun. 2022;626:44–50.
7. Gatt A, Agarwal S, Zito PM. Anatomy, Fascia Layers [Internet]. PubMed. Treasure Island (FL): StatPearls Publishing; 2020. Available from: https://www.ncbi.nlm.nih.gov/books/NBK526038/
8. Fede C, Pirri C, Fan C, Petrelli L, Guidolin D, De Caro R, et al. A closer look at the cellular and molecular components of the deep/muscular fasciae. Int J Mol Sci. 2021;22(3):1411.

9. Stecco C, Fede C, Macchi V, Porzionato A, Petrelli L, Biz C, et al. The fasciacytes: a new cell devoted to fascial gliding regulation. Clin Anat. 2018;31(5):667–76.
10. Dawidowicz J, Szotek S, Matysiak N, Mielańczyk Ł, Maksymowicz K. Electron microscopy of human fascia lata: focus on telocytes. J Cell Mol Med. 2015;19(10):2500–6.
11. Karamanos NK, Theocharis AD, Piperigkou Z, Manou D, Passi A, Skandalis SS, et al. A guide to the composition and functions of the extracellular matrix. The. FEBS J. 2021;288(24):6850.
12. Cabral-Pacheco GA, Garza-Veloz I, Castruita-De la Rosa C, Ramirez-Acuña JM, Perez-Romero BA, Guerrero-Rodriguez JF, et al. The roles of matrix metalloproteinases and their inhibitors in human diseases. Int J Mol Sci. 2020;21(24):9739.
13. Barber T, Esteban-Pretel G, Marín MP, Timoneda J. Vitamin A deficiency and alterations in the extracellular matrix. Nutrients. 2014;6(11):4984–5017.
14. Hodge C, Taylor C. Vitamin A deficiency [Internet]. PubMed. Treasure Island (FL): StatPearls Publishing; 2023. Available from: https://www.ncbi.nlm.nih.gov/books/NBK567744/
15. Cashman KD, Ritz C, Adebayo FA, Dowling KG, Itkonen ST, Öhman T, et al. Differences in the dietary requirement for vitamin D among Caucasian and east African women at northern latitude. Eur J Nutr. 2018;58(6):2281–91.
16. Pál É, Ungvári Z, Benyó Z, Várbíró S. Role of vitamin D deficiency in the pathogenesis of cardiovascular and cerebrovascular diseases. Nutrients. 2023;15(2):334.
17. Vy H, Nguyen YT, Kim N, Lee HJ. Vitamin A, D, E, and K as matrix metalloproteinase-2/9 regulators that affect expression and enzymatic activity. Int J Mol Sci. 2023;24(23):17038.
18. Miranpuri GS, Meethal SV, Sampene E, Chopra A, Buttar S, Nacht C, et al. Folic acid modulates matrix metalloproteinase-2 expression, alleviates neuropathic pain, and improves functional recovery in spinal cord-injured rats. Ann Neurosci. 2017;24(2):74–81.
19. Kendrová L, Mikuľáková W, Urbanová K, Andraščíková Š, Žultáková S, Takáč P, et al. Comprehensive decongestive therapy as a treatment for secondary lymphedema of the lower extremity and quality of life of women after gynecological cancer surgery. Med Sci Monit. 2020;26:e924071.
20. Poage EG, Rodrick JR, Wanchai A, Stewart BR, Cormier JN, Armer JM. Exploring the usefulness of botanicals as an adjunctive treatment for lymphedema: a systematic search and review. PM&R. 2014;7(3):296–310.
21. Singh B, Disipio T, Peake J, Hayes SC. Systematic review and meta-analysis of the effects of exercise for those with cancer-related lymphedema. Arch Phys Med Rehabil. 2016;97(2):302–15.

Hypofunction: Examples of Extracellular Matrix Involvement and Treatment

6

Aging can progress to the point of pathological findings and makes the development of various diseases more likely, but aging in itself is not, at first, a deep level of dysfunction. Aged ECM has a lack of functioning fibroblasts [1–4]. It has more senescence fibroblasts, which ought to have been replaced by more productive, newer, fibroblasts. If the ECM is an area of a basement membrane, then the laminin that connects the membrane to the matrix is reduced.

Proteins, ECM, and Aging

In this situation, decreased elastin and collagen in the ECM leads to less resistance to mechanical stressors. The structures of collagen observed in aging in the ECM are weaker, with less collagen overall and some crosslinking [4]. The crosslinked collagen has some resistance to stressors, but is not naturally formed. The crosslinking is often resulting from oxidative stress and glycation. As hyaluronic acid levels decrease, the ECM becomes less gel-like and hydrated, and stiffer. There are fewer fibroblasts, and some are senescent. The senescent fibroblasts are less productive and overall protein production is decreased. Basement membranes are weaker, and junctions in between cells are looser in

F. Smith, *The Extracellular Matrix in Health and Disease*,
https://doi.org/10.1007/978-3-031-94465-9_6

aging. This is partly due to less production of type IV collagen and most likely the anchoring proteoglycans (such as tensacin), which form these structures (Fig. 6.1).

Aging leads to a loss of total proteins in the matrisome. [1] This has been found to be true in animal models and human tissue assays. Moreover, inhibitory compounds such as lactadherin accumulate, although a paucity of lactadherin is found in hearts with accelerated aging and some pathological state (for instance, they have had one or more myocardial infarctions). This is found across ECM structural studies that production and inhibition need to be in balance for properly healthy function.

Appropriate turnover of proteins, including collagen, is important for normal ECM aging. Too much turnover will lead to degradation of the ECM and replacement with less organized, or excessively crosslinked collagen. Insufficient turnover leads to crosslinked collagen that has often accrued oxidative damage. In other words, excessively rapid repairs of matrix degradation and insufficient turnover of matrix can both result in an abnormal structure.

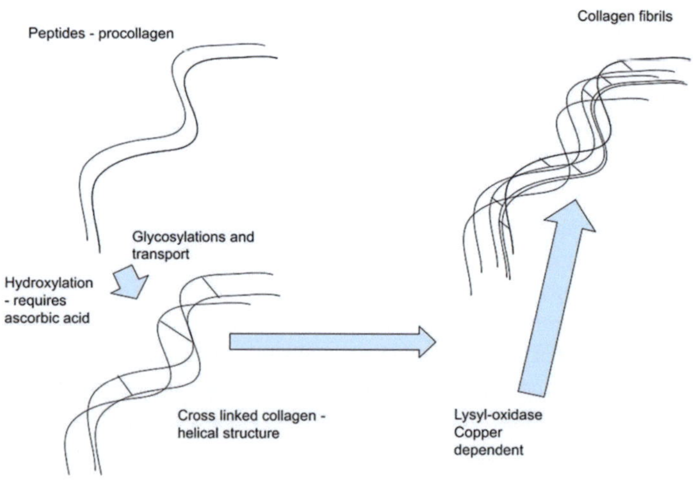

Fig. 6.1 Extracellular matrix in hypofunction

The ECM Is Not Only Impacted by Aging, but Determines It to an Extent

In animal models, and in observations of humans, the ECM changes with age. Fibroblasts are less numerous, and as mentioned, become senescent. Collagen becomes more crosslinked, and the matrix becomes stiffer. Elastin becomes fragmented, in spite of its decades-long life. The changes to the ECM lead to changes in mechanotransduction. This has an effect, via the connections to cell membrane integrin and C44, on the transcription of genes in the surrounding cells. In experimental models, when the cells of a younger organism are placed into aged ECM, they quickly show signs of dysfunction. Conversely, when senescent cells, including stem cells, are placed into the ECM from a younger organism, they exhibit increased ability to renew themselves and to create normal tissue structures. Mesenchymal stem cells in a younger ECM are more reparative. In the aged ECM, stem cells are actually inhibited [5].

Elastin

Humans form almost all of their elastin during the prenatal and infancy periods of development. Elastin is formed from tropoelastin precursors, which are rich in hydrophobic amino acids such as proline. These monomer precursors are woven together with microfibrillar proteins to make elastic fibers. This is a complete formation process and does not really happen after the neonatal period.

Elastin can be broken down by elastase enzymes, which can happen during remodeling after injury (Fig. 6.2). The collagen that takes its place or other ECM proteins will be structurally strong but lack the property of elasticity. Elastin fibers give tissues, both larger structural ones such as the outer vascular wall, and the pervasive ECM, the ability to absorb stress by stretching, and to return that energy to the tissue. This leads to flexibility and rapid recovery from deformation to the body. In the case of the arteries, it also means that kinetic energy from the bloodstream

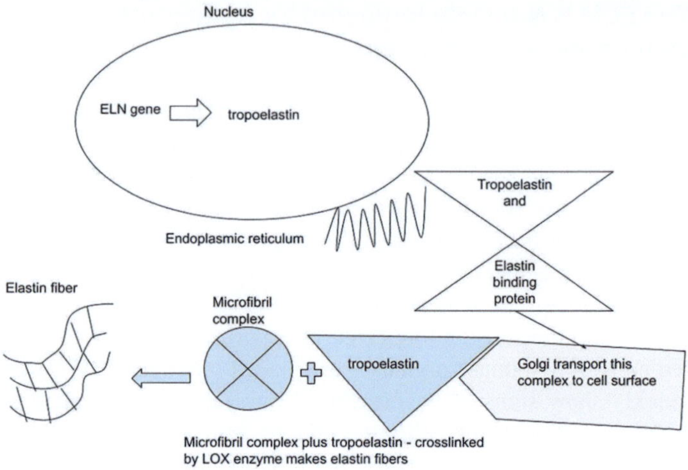

Fig. 6.2 Elastin formation

that is channeled into elastic arteries will be absorbed by those arterial walls and returned to the circulatory flow. This not only gives compliance to the artery (which reduces the peripheral resistance to ventricular ejection of blood) but provides a return of the energy to help propel the blood forward in the circuit [6, 7].

Elastin found in the arteries is a good cxample of the importance of this protein. It is found in various levels of the arterial wall (Fig. 6.3). These tissues contain elastin both in specialized layers of the artery, and within the arterial ECM. As mentioned, elastases can degrade elastin, and this can happen due to excessive oxidative stress, damage due to shearing forces in the artery (especially in conditions of elevated blood pressure), and advanced glycation end products (which are elevated in conditions of inflammation, higher oxidative stress, and blood glucose, as one might see in the pervasive metabolic syndrome).

Elastase activity is found in neutrophils that produce elastases (hence the importance of local injury and the response to it, which often involve white blood cell migration to the area), and matrix metalloproteinases. When elastin is degraded, it produces elastin-derived peptides. Not only can these be used as a marker of elastin

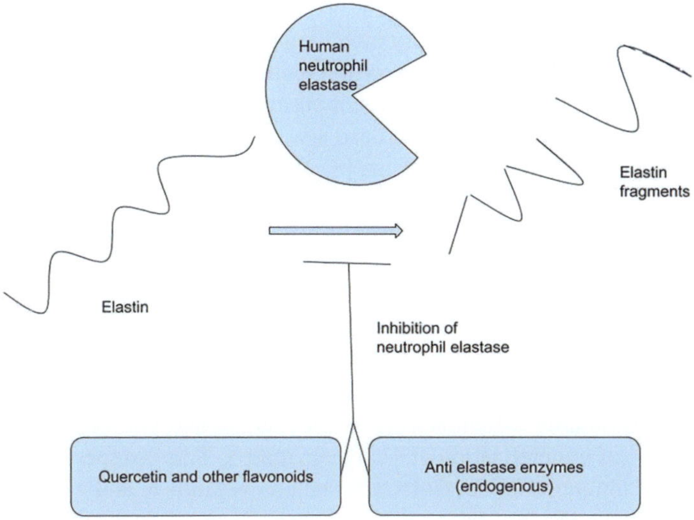

Fig. 6.3 Elastase and anti-elastase

destruction, but the elastin-derived peptides can bind to specific receptors, the elastin receptor complex (ERC). This causes a series of reactions, mediated by Neu-1 subunit of the ERC. The downstream effects include activation of protein kinases and extracellular matrix remodeling. This is a pathway to a stiffer, more aged, ECM.

The effects of loss of elastin in the lung are well known and exemplified by the emphysema form of chronic obstructive pulmonary disease (but certainly not limited to this presentation). In the case of emphysema with an etiology of smoking, the repeated bursts of oxidative stress and direct damage from tobacco smoke (with too many noxious compounds to itemize here) lead to a practicable response to injury. Neutrophil elastases degrade alveolar walls in the lung and surround ECM. Those with an inherent deficiency of *anti*-elastase proteins are going to suffer more damage. The oxidants and toxins in the cigarette smoke actually disable some of the anti-elastases, which of course makes matters worse. Over time, the lungs lose their elastic recoil, and the person will develop an inflated thorax with increased AP diameter, and hypertrophied accessory breathing muscles (and the architectural changes to the thorax will eventually inhibit normal diaphragmatic function). This loss of elasticity, coupled with loss of alveolar walls and increased dead spaces in the lungs, will create the disease state of emphysema [8, 9].

Bone and Weak ECM

Osteoporosis is a common condition that becomes more prevalent with age, found in both males and females. Bone density peaks at maturity, and then slowly declines. The formation of hydroxyapatite, which is made from calcium and phosphate, is a source of mineralization of a collagen matrix. This is a specialized ECM unique to bone. Cofactors such as vitamin K and zinc are also needed for this process. Defective ECM due to lack of protein in the diet, and simple dissolution of the ECM with aging, means that bone quality will decrease as well. Joint tissue is lined with cartilage, which is a specialized tissue of condensed ECM. Hyaline, elastic, and fibrillar cartilage differ in their collagen density, but all cartilage contains this protein, plus proteoglycans [5].

Advanced Glycation End Products and Collagen Crosslinking

There are two major pathways of extracellular crosslinking of collagen. Collagen fibrils start out as triple-helical proteins in the cell, and this is facilitated by hydroxylation of protein with vitamin C and iron as some of the cofactors. Once excreted into the ECM, they become woven together as triple helices. Lysyl oxidase (LOX) is a key enzyme in the ECM. It produces aldehydes, allysine, and hydroxylysine made from deamination of lysine and hydroxylysine. These form weak crosslinks, which can become sturdier, and more permanent covalent crosslinks. This is what makes collagen strong and provides the scaffolding for many body tissues [10].

The other crosslinking pathway is that of glycation. This is the modification of a protein by reaction with a reducing sugar. These sugars include glucose, fructose, pentoses, galactose, mannose, and xylulose. Although many proteins in the body, including the proteins of the matrix, have glycation aspects, there is a pathological type of glycation that hinders normal function. But some glycations are abnormal and essentially disable proteins due to their conjugation with advanced glycation end products (AGEs).

AGEs are well known in cooking, for example, braising meat creates the Maillard reaction, which leads to a flavorful and crispy texture. Many people are now aware that hemoglobin A1C is a diagnostic and monitoring test for diabetes. Reducing sugars can produce advanced glycation end products via several pathways. A common route is for an initial condensation reaction to form a Schiff base, followed by a rearrangement to create Amadori products, which can release alpha-dicarbonyl compounds (glyoxyl, methylglyoxyl), which can bind to proteins and crosslink proteins together. The alpha-dicarbonyl pathways can also be formed directly from the Schiff base through what is called the Namiki pathway. Reducing sugars can also become alpha-dicarbonyls through autooxidation, which are iron and copper catalyzed, known as the Wolff pathway. The polyol pathway, via an initial conversion to frucrose-6-phosphate, can produce alpha di-carbonyls. The glycolytic pathway can lead straight to advanced glycation end products (AGE) via glyceraldehyde 3 phosphate and fructose-6-phosphate [10].

This biochemical pathway is damaging to the extracellular matrix. The excessive crosslinking of collagen leads to a loss of functionality of the ECM. The increased stiffness interferes with the mechanotransduction functions of the ECM. This has effects on cellular proliferation, gene expression, autophagy, and migration. This kind of degraded ECM is also suppressive to local stem cells, such that the capacity of the tissue in question to regenerate itself is diminished. It contributes to a tumor-permissive environment. It is also a pathway to states of chronic inflammation. Damage to the microvascular system, which is strongly accelerated by ECM damage, leads to increased risk of cardiovascular disease. Many diabetic complications are strongly driven by the presence of AGE and polyols.

Senescence-Associated Secretory Phenotype (SASP)

As cells age, they change their phenotypic expression. In the ECM, fibroblasts will replace themselves normally in youth, and as aging progresses, they are slower to do so. The accumulation of senescent fibroblasts means a reduction in collagen formation. Older collagen that has less turnover may become crosslinked [11]. The ECM in aging shows more secretion of soluble factors [matrix metalloproteinases (MMPs)], growth factors, and angiogenic factors. The macrophages and neutrophils in the SASP are likely to be polarized to M2 and N2 subtypes. These are anti-inflammatory, which has some benefits, but they are less able to stop tumor cells and more likely to become tumor-associated (allied to cancer cells), should a neoplasm arise.

Hypofunction in General

Changes to the ECM that lead to hypofunction can be aging-related, but they can occur earlier in life as well. For example, a diet rich in fructose and oxidized fatty acids and deficient in protein will compromise ECM stability in a younger individual. Exposure to toxins will likewise degrade collagen structure and create elastase fragments. For example, polyethylene microplastics (which are unfortunately ubiquitous) can embed in the ECM, disrupt its function, and disrupt normal signaling of the innate immune system. This is just one example of toxic disruption—there are thousands of environmental toxins. Some are naturally occurring and others are available due to human deposition (such as mercury, which is an element, but is found in the food webs of the planet mostly due to human contamination). Many chemical compounds have been synthesized in the last 100 years. Millions of compounds have been synthesized in labs, but only some are used for any purpose in the world. The number of compounds that have been synthesized and put into commercial or industrial use is often cited as 100,000. Research in this decade suggests that this number is a large underestimate—and that the number may be closer to 350,000. Some may be inert or nontoxic, others are known to be toxic, and many others are still a mystery as to what their true and long-term effects on humans are [12].

The exposure of toxins that damage the ECM can give rise to disease. It also leads to less function in general, even when disease symptoms or the progression of pathology have not yet occurred. The ECM functions of mechanotransduction that impact cellular genetic expression, proliferation, and migration are impaired. This makes for a less resilient tissue or organ, and gives way to a phenotype that is ripe for deeper dysfunction.

Therapeutic Considerations

Therapy is very rooted in ensuring that the determinant factors of the requirements of health are being met, which is the hallmark of naturopathic medicine. Specific to ECM support, the diet needs to have sufficient amino acids and cofactors for proper protein (collagen especially) formation. This is discussed below. Additionally, the limitation of exposure to toxins that degrade the ECM is important. The buttressing of antioxidant enzyme systems and dietary antioxidants are important preserving factors for the ECM. Ultimately, the goal is to prevent the development of a phenotype that can prematurely age and become inflammatory, or especially, tumor permissive [13].

Anti-Elastase and Collagenase Plant Extracts

Camellia sinensis, the tea plant, yields a number of compounds that can reduce elastase and collagenase activity. White tea and green tea are very similar, but have slightly different processing. There are also different varieties and countries of origin (e.g., China, Japan, Sri Lanka) of green and white tea. White tea is picked from smaller buds of the tea plant, with silver or white fibers (or "hairs") around the bud. It is very minimally processed, usually some outdoor sun drying on bamboo holders with temperature and humidity controlled indoor drying to follow. Green tea, by contrast, is gently heated through steaming or an iron pan. Drying in either case leads to some oxidation, but many of the compounds of the plant remain intact [14].

Camellia sinensis has the following compounds of note:

Polyphenols include catechins, flavonoids, anthocyanins, and phenolic acids.

Catechins include epicatechin and epicatechin 3 gallate. These molecules are potent antioxidants and have anticancer functions as well.

Flavonoids include flavonol glycosides such as quercetin, which has an array of anti-inflammatory and antitumor actions.

Anthocyanins are plant pigments and are large aggregates of phenolic molecules. They have both antioxidant and collagen-stabilizing functions. They are not as concentrated in tea as the catechins.

Phenolic compounds such as chlorogenic, gallic, and ellagic acid contribute to the antioxidant functions of tea.

Alkaloids

Alkaloids are nitrogenous compounds that usually have an interaction with the human nervous system. These bitter compounds are well known as some of the important medicinal compounds, such as morphine, nicotine, and colchicine. The alkaloids in tea are caffeine, theophylline, and theobromine. These compounds are competitive antagonists to adenosine, which can cause modulation in excitatory neurotransmitters, such as increased norepinephrine(adenosine being a naturally produce relaxant that slows heart rate). They are well-known antifatigue (at least as a primary effect) compounds since by blocking adenosine, caffeine, and the other methylxanthines, they delay the perception of tiredness and can help maintain mental stamina (keeping in mind that a secondary effect of being more fatigued will result in time). Theophylline is an asthma medicine that can act as a bronchodilator by relaxing the muscles of the airway. It is also useful in asthma since the adenosine antagonism reduces the release of histamine by blocking cAMP mechanisms. While these alkaloids and their functions in higher amounts can have an inhibitory effect on ECM production, they tend to be in lower amounts (compared to black tea and coffee, another methylxanthine source) [14].

Epigallocatechine gallate is available as a dietary supplement, and while not possessing the entire range of flavonoids, phenols, and catechins, it does have potent antioxidant and antitumor (in the microenvironment activity) effects. This also eliminates methylxanthine intake. Nevertheless, dietary consumption of green, or white, tea seems safe for the ECM, as does moderate intake of yellow, oolong, and black tea. These teas are more oxidized, which reduces catchin activity but produces theaflavin, which inhibits degradation of the ECM. This certainly underscores the value of plant beverages that offset caffeine with a variety of compounds, versus widely consumed soft drinks that have added caffeine but no beneficial compounds.

Polyphenols, which are abundant in the tea plant, but found in many plant sources, are not only antioxidants but can non covalently crosslinked collagen. That is, they can cause reversible but stabilizing molecular bridges between collagen fibrils, which strengthens the structures of the ECM. This is in contrast to the covalent crosslinks that we see in scar tissue, and in the tumor microenvironment. Those crosslinks, when too prevalent, can lead to a stiffening of the ECM, which creates a host of problems. One of the maladaptations of excessive crosslinking is that the mechanotransduction functions of the ECM are impaired, with still being discovered effects on cell replication and migration.

Polyphenols are excellent antioxidants, but like most acceptors of free radicals, they can become oxidizing molecules under certain conditions. For polyphenols, it appears that metal-catalyzed reactions, such as an environment with excessive iron, can yield polyphenols that act as prooxidants that can interact with other molecules. This can include modulation of the lysine residues on some proteins. This underscores the importance of optimal functioning of the body's intrinsic enzyme system for control of oxidative stress. Enzymes such as superoxide dismutase and glutathione synthase/glutathione reductase must be functioning in order to maximize the benefits of dietary polyphenols.

Ferroptosis is the destruction of cells, including ECM structures and cells, in an iron-catalyzed pathway. The iron element acts as a catalyst for rapid free radical propagation. This is a cause of some cellular necrosis, upregulation of inflammation, and damage to elastin fibers. A useful plant to negate ferroptosis is *Hippophae rhamnoides* or sea buckthorn. This is a plant from traditional Tibetan medicine. It is a hardy plant that can grow in poor or salty soils (such as near an ocean coastline), and withstand very cold temperatures. It contains flavonoids such as isorhamnetin, kaempferol, and quercetin, triterpenoid saponins, as well as proanthocyanidins. It can have vascular supportive functions, in addition to some ability to suppress ferroptosis.

Chondroitin Sulfate

This molecule is a glycosaminoglycan found throughout the ECM. It is composed of repeating units of sugars; (N-acetylgalactosamine and glucuronic acid). It can be found bonded to a protein to make a proteoglycan. It is an important part of cartilage. Chondroitin sulfate as a supplement gained some popularity starting in the 1990s for osteoarthritis. Although it will improve joint lubrication and reduce pain, its actual use goes beyond providing precursors for cartilage formation. It appears to help rebuild the ECM in general. It also decreases localized inflammation. It is well absorbed, which might require some digestive action to break some of the bonds in the repeating sugar chain. Human doses of 4000 mg per day seem to be most effective.

Chondroitin sulfate in biological models of senescence and longevity resources appears to increase lifespan. To whatever degree it does this for humans, it may be due to its ability to improve ECM homeostasis [15].

Metformin

Metformin (dimethylbiguanide) is a widely used drug for the treatment of diabetes mellitus, particularly non-insulin-dependent diabetes mellitus. It increases the sensitivity of muscle cells to insulin. It was originally derived from the herbal medicine *Galega officinalis*

(Goat's rue). Metformin activates AMP-activated protein kinase (AMPK), which leads to lower blood sugar levels and overall better function of the GLUT-4 transporter. Metformin also appears to modulate matrix metalloproteinase activity and reduce TGF-beta, leading to a more stable ECM. Metformin is a complete mode of action, with several pathways to impact MAPK and other effects on the functions of the mitochondria and on the enzymes of the liver. Although drug prescriptions are not the starting point of naturopathic medicine, this is a widely used medicine that is available to naturopathic physicians to use in some jurisdictions. The fact that it can preserve ECM integrity and reduce excessive inflammatory enzyme destruction of the matrix is worth noting in the sense of optimizing ECM function. This is also relevant for those to whom metformin is often prescribed—diabetics. Their ECM proteins are susceptible to crosslinking by advanced glycation end products, and the self-propagating oxidative reactions can age the ECM in diabetics [16].

Arctium lappa (Burdock) This plant is used in herbal medicine to encourage biliary drainage and for its traditional use for various skin eruptions such as psoriasis. *Arctium lappa* has polyphenols, much like green tea (*Camellia sinensis*), including gallic acid and chlorogenic acid. These are anti-elastase and can help preserve the important elastin content of the ECM, which is not really replaced with age. *Arctium lappa* also contains arctigenin, a compound that can upregulate AMP-activated protein kinase. This has a direct anti-elastase effect. It also can prevent excessive collagen deposition. This has implications for the prevention of fibrosis and the modulation of the tumor microenvironment, topics that are addressed in later chapters of this book. As a side note, *Arctium lappa* can also increase cyclic adenosine monophosphate (cAMP) in cells, which has other effects such as regulated cell turnover [17].

Sleep, Daylight Exposure, and Circadian Rhythms

Circadian systems work in a chronological fashion. Daylight is an important clock setter with regards to the pituitary via inputs to the retina and signals sent via the retinal-hypothalamic tract. This central clock can synchronize with tissue and organ-specific clocks. This time-keeping system has an enormous influence on the extracellular matrix. The formation and degradation of collagen, as well as the release of signaling proteoglycans, is rhythmic and under circadian control. This is an example of a major biogregulatory system influencing the ECM.

The ECM itself has a bioregulatory function with regards to the greater circadian control systems. The localized circadian clocks work optimally in a healthy (and younger) extracellular matrix. In a stiff, crosslinked, and aged ECM, these zeitgebers (timegivers) become erratic and/or out of sync with the central clock. This can also pull that organ or tissue out of synchronization with hormone levels, notably cortisol. Conversely, the biochemical and biomechanical properties of the ECM influence the strength of circadian rhythm in a cell type-specific manner. During aging, the ECM properties are altered and the circadian clocks are dampened, leading to irregular sleep/wake cycle, dampening, and misalignment of circadian rhythms in body temperature and hormone levels.

For this reason, circadian regularity is of the utmost importance to prevent hypofunction of the ECM. The necessity of sleep and its deprivation are well known. Cardiovascular, immune, and CNS issues galore can arise from lack of sleep and disturbed circadian rhythms. But the maintenance of a healthy ECM (which leads to homeostasis of the local tissues) is dependent on the proper function of the central and peripheral circadian systems [18].

Sleep hygiene is a well-known aid in this regard, but often ignored. Regular bedtimes, reduction in screen time before bed, avoidance of excessive sugar, caffeine, and food with several hours of retirement, are all important. A quiet, dark, well-ventilated, and temperature-optimized (cool but this has variation among people) sleep environment is important.

Melatonin is useful for those who have a dysregulated photo-retinal-hypothalamic-pituitary system, such as shift workers and long-distance travelers [19]. Magnesium malate can be helpful as magnesium is a muscle relaxant that many adults lack. There are a host of nervine/ sedative/hypnotic botanicals that can be useful judiciously to help normalize sleep–wake cycles. The idea of using an herbal preparation is not to become dependent on it to sleep. It is best used to re-establish a healthy regimen that will continue on its own [20].

Tightly Bound Water, Aging, and Tissue Stiffness

As humans age, their tissues become less able to bind water at the ECM level. To a large degree, this is due to excessive crosslinking of the covalent kind and the accumulation (which increases the crosslinking) of advanced glycation end products. This contributes to a state of dehydration in a specific way. When water binds to glycoproteins in the ECM, it becomes a plasticizer. The matrix at that point, and therefore the tissues as a whole, becomes more plastic, flexible, and better able to conduct mechanotransduction duties. As people age, the tissues and the ECM are less able to bind water to the glycoproteins and the ECM reflects that issue in becoming even more rigid. This hastens aging and causes a general loss of efficiency of basic biological processes. It also has visible effects on vascular compliance, which can be measured by changes in blood pressure and peripheral arterial resistance. But the same phenomenon of stiffness, due to a lack of bound water, is an organism-wide phenomenon as we age [21].

Many of the aforementioned therapies are de-stiffening agents. Polyphenols, flavonoids, vitamin D, and ascorbic acid are all useful. Tissue-specific de-stiffening agents tend to have more tissue-specific bioflavonoids, such as the case where silymarin flavonolignans from *Silybum marianum* (Milk thistle) have a liver, and kidney, antifibrotic effect [22]. But even below the threshold of fibrosis, there is a precursor of stiffening due to loss of elastin, and importantly, bound water.

Dietary Amino Acids

The intake of amino acids across the world varies depending on cultural and cuisine practices, and socioeconomic factors [23]. In North America, although hunger is on the rise, there are many people who consume adequate or even excessive protein. In terms of percentage of caloric intake, the intake is about 15% of total kCal. Like all tissues, the ECM has protein turnover as a result of enzymatic remodeling, which includes the breakdown of damaged proteins. Adequate dietary protein to stay in nitrogen balance is supportive of collagen and the ECM [24, 25].

Taurine, carnosine, and other amino acids from meat are supportive of some connective tissues, the retina, and the heart and other muscles. Taurine can be synthesized from cysteine but dietary intakes are helpful in optimizing levels. Nonmeat eaters can supplement taurine if this is indicated as can those who have animal proteins in their diet. Sulfur intake is supportive of proper cartilage formation. Overabundance of sulfur in some disease states can lead to problems, such as hepatic fibrosis [26].

Exercise

Exercise reconditions the ECM in multiple ways. A remarkable systematic review by Kritikaki et al. (2021) looked at multiple exercise studies and the effect on muscle extracellular matrix [27]. These studies involved different age groups and different types and duration of exercise training. In addition to the expected results of better strength, aerobic capacity, and faster results in the young, the studies showed that exercise increases the expression of mRNA and proteins that make up the ECM. This includes the many types of collagens in the muscle ECM, fibronectin, laminin, and others. This review provides very detailed information about many studies that used different exercise approaches, but the overall effect appears to be an increase in ECM construction. Although this is focused on muscle tissue, this type of tissue is about a third of the total body mass. The powerful MoTrPAC Study Group published a sweeping analysis of exercise effects on the whole organism, including cellular components such as mitochondria [28]. Extracellular matrix is included in these overall effects, including the remodeling to become less thick in some cases of endurance training.

Regulating Oxidative Activity

Free radicals are a normal aspect of biological systems, but if not adequately controlled they can cause tissue damage, inflammation, and genetic mutations. The support of antioxidant systems goes beyond the extracellular matrix and includes mitochondria, cell membrane, cytoplasm, organelles, and nucleus. However, oxidative damage to the ECM can contribute to inflammation and maladaptive remodeling [29, 30]. Enzymatic and nonenzymatic crosslinking can become excessive after repeated injury. This can lead to a stiffening of the matrix, which has the effect of accelerating aging.

Nutritional cofactors such as alpha-lipoic acid and carotenoids are important as circulating antioxidants. Vital to the regulation of antioxidant function, as mentioned, are the basic enzymatic systems that protect ECM-cellular units of life.

Superoxide dismutase is a key enzyme that changes an oxygen radical (which will always be present in the body due to both aerobic metabolism and external stressors that act as oxidants) to H2O2 (hydrogen peroxide). It has zinc, copper, and manganese forms, with manganese (Mn) being important for SOD2, a key antioxidant in mitochondria. This hydrogen peroxide is converted by the enzyme catalase to water and oxygen in its stable doublet form [31].

The intracellular enzyme glutathione peroxidase-1 can turn hydrogen peroxide into water. The oxidized by-product can be restored to a useful form by the enzyme glutathione reductase. Nutritional requirements for glutathione include amino acids, particularly cysteine, selenium, vitamin C, and some B vitamins such as riboflavin and methylfolate [32, 33].

Dietary antioxidants can have a glutathione-sparing function by nonenzymatically absorbing an unpaired electron. These antioxidants often contain a phenol group, but isoprenoids are also good at absorbing a free radical. People who consume not only a nutrient-dense diet, but one with enough plant foods, will tend to have a good supply of these antioxidants. Those who consume a lot of burnt or deep-fried foods will add to their general level of oxidative stress because these foods also contain free radical propagators, such as hydroperoxides from fryer oil, and heterocyclic amines and polycyclic aromatic hydrocarbons from burnt (or extreme temperature cooked) foods.

Detoxification

The aforementioned nutrients that support antioxidant enzymes and have direct antioxidant activity are useful in the biotransformation of xenobiotics, including those that are toxic to humans at some threshold. These antioxidants can be helpful as bystanders that protect tissues, particularly the hepatocytes, during biotransformation using a sequence of cytochrome P450 mixed-function oxidases that make a toxin initially reactive, followed by conjugation to a secondary molecule that renders the product inert and water soluble. These steps are sometimes called phases 1 and 2. Glutathione itself can become a conjugate during phase 2 as can amino acids, glucuronic acid, sulfate, acetyl, and methyl groups.

In addition to this important central detoxification, there is the matter of toxin deposition and retention in the extracellular matrix. For example, glyphosate (sold as "Round Up" in the United States) is an herbicide that is ubiquitous. This compound can substitute for the amino acid glycine in the proteoglycans in the ECM, as well as in collagen. Thus, the ECM can act as a reservoir for these substances. The precise health consequences of this sequestration of glyphosate and the degree of exposure required to create disease are under scientific investigation, but this serves as an example of how the ECM can trap toxins.

Fluoroquinolones, a class of widely used and powerful antibiotics, are known to cause tendinopathies, including Achilles tendon rupture. This is due to the actions of the drug in the ECM of the tendon. Signaling molecules that could lead to growth and repair of the collagen in the tendon are suppressed, and matrix metalloproteinases are activated, which can cause weakening of the collagen structures. This does not negate the overall usefulness of this class of drugs, but illustrates much the ECM can be influenced by a drug.

Mercury is a heavy metal that is found throughout the world due to soil and water contamination. It is used in electrical transmission equipment and in the past was used medicinally as mercury chloride (HgCl2). Mercury in the form of methylmercury (HgCH4) from fish, as well as ethylmercury (fish and vaccinations, which contain about the same amount of Hg++ as a meal of tuna) and mercury vapor (from dental amalgams), can be absorbed and deposit in the matrix and damage tissues. This leads to inflammatory reactions. In the vascular wall, this can lead to overactivate fibroblasts and growth of atheromatous plaques. In the brain, this leads to increased oxidative stress, glutamate excitotoxicity, and neuroinflammation [34].

Hormesis

Hormesis is the phenomenon of low-dose biological stressors leading to adaptive changes in the organism. The concept of low doses of a substance leads to adaptive responses, whereas that same substance could be a toxin at higher amounts. This was in sense proposed by the physician Paracelsus and others. In the late nineteenth and early twentieth centuries, the work of pharmacologists Arndt and Schultz led to a principle named after them. This Arndt–Schultz principle stated that low doses of a substance could stimulate and high doses inhibit. They described a diphasic dose–response curve. The idea that the stimulatory zone, while not overly forceful, could lead to adaptive changes in the organism got some study, but as the twentieth century moved on; this area of Hormesis (from the Greek word "to excite") began to languish. Some midcentury interest in radiation hormesis created scientific interest, but hormesis did not progress as a project commensurate with its great potential for explaining the ways in which biological systems respond to low-dose stimuli including medicines.

The professor of pharmacology at the University of Massachusetts, Dr. Edward Calabrese, reignited interest in hormesis and truly articulated the concept in terms of modern pharmacological sciences [35–37]. Starting in the 1990s, Calabrese took time to develop this through many bioassays, which involved more sensitive, broader, and finer measurements of responses. Moreover, they included pharmacologists in this discussion via collaborative work, symposia, and publication in respected journals. In the following 30 years, hormesis research has advanced incredibly.

According to Calabrese, the hormetic response is about halfway (on the dose–response curve) between zero, and that point at which we might see observable adverse effects. This is a subthreshold as far as true toxicity and in terms of what a drug might be considered to do in its effective dose. For about a third of substances including drugs, there is a response in the hormetic zone that is opposite the effect in the more linear dose–response curve further on. For example, a drug that causes death of tumor cells in its typical higher dose use can cause tumor proliferation in the hormetic zone. This is a biphasic response. The magnitude of this response, as well articulated by Calabrese, is about 150% of controls. So, it is significant, but modest. It does not imbalance the organism.

This becomes medically interesting in a few ways. For one, hormetic responses are a fact of life, so knowing the potential for biphasic responses is important to give precise treatment. Cannabidiol (CBD) is a compound from *Cannabis sativa* that many people use for pain, restlessness, and sleeplessness. CBD has a biphasic response curve, and increasing doses are less effective outside of the top of that response.

Hormesis research has led to a highly relevant and promising body of research. If low-dose stimuli can cause mild stress to the organism, which leads to adaptive responses via expression of certain genes, then intentionally giving low-dose stimuli that cause a safe challenge to the organism can lead to that organism becoming stronger. This has implications for improved metabolism, resilience, cancer prevention, and decelerated aging.

One example of a hormetic action relative to the ECM is that of induction of NRF2 (nuclear factor erythroid 2-related factor 2). NRF2 is held in the cytosol by KEAP (Kelch-like ECH-associated protein 1). Oxidative causes KEAP to "let go" of NRF2, from which point NRF 2 goes to the nucleus and binds to the antioxidant response element (ARE). This response element "turns on" phase 2 genes, which leads to increases in glutathione and other molecules that can intercept oxidative stress.

In addition to true oxidative stress, plant compounds such as sulforaphane from cruciferous vegetables (broccoli, brussels sprouts, etc.) can cause KEAP to release NRF2 with the result of increased antioxidant defenses. The plant extracts in any kind of dietary amount are not harmful, they simply provide a small stressor to the cell—"as if" there were free radicals or electrophilic molecules in the area. This uptick in antioxidant production can protect the proteins, glycoproteins, sugars, and other molecules of the ECM from oxidative damage.

Mitohormesis is a type of hormetic responsiveness that opens up adaptive changes in the mitochondria [38–40]. This is a conserved response across multiple species across time. One form of stress on the mitochondria is the stiffening of the ECM as is the often-related glycation of ECM proteins. Mitochondria adapt via several pathways, and one is the heat shock protein 1 (HSF1), which starts a process that increases two other transcription factors (e.g., RPN4 and PDR3). These responses lead to an increase in protein chaperone activity that benefits the mitochondria. Many mitochondrial proteins are actually assembled in the cytosol by ribosomes and then imported back into the mitochondria. These responses to HSF1 and its effectors also lead to better clearance of damaged proteins in the mitochondria. This is done by ubiquitination whereby a senescence or damaged protein is tagged with several ubiquitin proteins that lead to its destruction in the proteasome. This essentially clears molecular garbage from the mitochondria (Fig. 6.4).

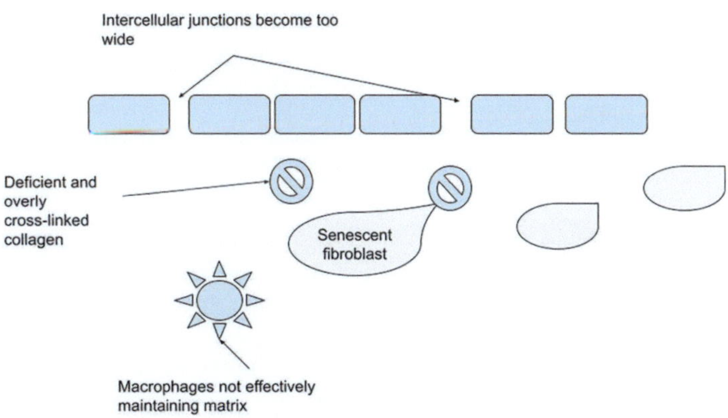

Fig. 6.4 Hypofunction in ECM

Berberine is an alkaloid found in plants such as *Hydrastis canadensis* and *Mahonia (Berberis) aqualfolia*. Berberine is an inducer of mitohormesis via upregulation of MAPK (5′ adenosine monophosphate-activated protein kinase). It can do this right in the mitochondria after entry into the organelle via the organic cation transporter on the mitochondrial membrane. MAPK activation increases autophagy and increases the number of mitochondria in the cell. In the sense of general hypofunction of the ECM, hormetic approaches can be considered to upregulate protein synthesis.

Therapies to reduce collagen and elastin destruction [41–46]

Therapy	Mechanism	Dose	Remarks
EGCG epigallocatechin gallate [14]	Inhibits elastase; absorbs oxidative stress	200–400 mg per day	Can be obtained from tea—*Camelia sinensis* (less oxidized teas such as green and white tea have higher EGCG levels)
Galium aparine (cleavers) [45]	Flavonoids and phenols inhibit elastase	Tincture (ethanol–water extract) 5 ml 1× or 2× per day Dried herb: 500 mg 1× or 2× per day	Gallium aparine has a traditional medicine use of activating lymph flow
Arcitum lappa (burdock) [14]	Polyphenolic compounds in roots inhibit elastase	Tincture (ethanol–water extract) 3 ml 2× per day or 3× per day Dried root—1 g 1× per day or 2× per day	The whole plant including leaves can be consumed but root preparations are more common. This plant has the ability to encourage the flow of bile from the hepatobilliary tract

Therapy	Mechanism	Dose	Remarks
Fucus vesiculosis (and other *Fucus* species) (kelp; Bladdewrack) [14]	The polysaccharides (such as fucoidan) and phlorotanins (a phenolic compound found in marine plants) inhibit elastase	500 mg encapsulation 1× per day or 2× per day (but higher amounts can be consumed as kelp is a safe food)	Used as a source of iodine and has benefits in diabetes
Luteolin (flavonoid) [47]	Inhibits neutrophil elastase	300 mg per day Also found in many plants such as *Taraxacum officinale* (dandelion) and *Ligustrum lucidum* (privet)	Given the inhibition of neutrophil elastase
Hippophae rhamnoides (sea buckthorn) [43, 44]	Contains isorhamnetin, kaempferol, and quercetin, triterpenoid saponins, which block inflammatory destruction of proteins	500 mg sea Buckthorne oil bid	Many cardiovascular and ECM protective benefits

Therapies to reduce excessive collagen covalent crosslinking and to increase ECM water binding

Therapy	Mechanism	Dose	Remarks
EGCG epigallocatechin gallate [14]	Anti-collagenase activity	200–400 mg per day	As noted above, also inhibit elastase
Withania somnifera (Ashwagandha) [48]	Withanolides (a series of similar steroidal compounds) can prevent free radical-induced covalent crosslinking of collagen	500 mg 2× per day 3 ml of tincture (ethanol–water extract) 2× per day	In addition to this ECM protective function, *Withania somnifera* has many adaptogenic (anti-fatigue, immune and mental support) functions
Proanthocyanidins including extract of *Vaccinium myrtillus* [49]	While these complex flavonoid structures can reinforce collagen fibrils, they have very strong antioxidant ability and can prevent the excessive covalent crosslinking of collagen	Bilberry extract (*Vaccinium myrtillus*) 500 mg 2× per day	Adding berries (blueberries, raspberries, blackberries, thimbleberries, huckleberries, mulberries) to the diet each day can provide these compounds

Therapies to regulate circadian rhythms

Therapy	Mechanism	Dose	Remarks
Exercise [50]	Multiple: Hormetic effects but also increases in microcirculation, mobilization of fascia, and increases in collagen	Highly individualized—Should include strength, flexibility, aerobic, and agility aspects Per doctor's recommendation	At minimum, CDC recommendation of 150 min of moderate-intensity exercise per week (adults) and 2 sessions of muscle-strengthening activity per week
Sleep duration and quality [50]	In order for normal night-time functions (such as glymphatic system discharge from the brain, growth hormone secretion by the pituitary, CREB protein in the brain to encode learning) to execute the person must obtain some deeper levels of sleep	Varies per person (https://www.cdc.gov/sleep/about/index.html) states that adults 18–65 need at least 7 h per night	Quality can be impacted by many health issues from apnea, or sinus and septal issues, heart disease, pain, etc
Sunlight exposure [51]	Sets the retinohypothalamic tract—And the master clock for all circadian rhythms	Daylight exposure beginning early and with additional exposures—Does not have to be direct sunlight	Lighting in the home, screens, and ambient lighting in the community (streetlights), and staying indoors can impact this cycle

Therapies that help to include a functional ECM phenotype including hormetins

Therapy	Mechanism	Dose or activity	Remarks
Sulforaphane [52]	NRF2 activator	6 mg per day (this is usually presented on supplement facts labels as a sulforaphane yield from a precursor such as a broccoli extract)	Foods are an excellent source of this compound, particularly (cruciferous vegetables: Broccoli, cauliflowers, cabbage, kale, Brussels sprouts, arugula, bok choy, collard greens, radishes, turnips, and watercress)
Curcumin [53]	NRF 2 activator and NFKbeta inhibition	600 mg of curcumin per day Curcmin bound to phosphatidyl choline (phytosome) will have better absorption Higher amounts can be used	Curcmin may also be packaged as mixed curcuminoids (similar compounds): Curcumin, demethoxycurcumin, bisdemethoxycurcumin
Resveratrol [54]	NRF2 activator and works against excessive collagen crosslinking	200 mg or 400 mg per day depending on level of oxidative stress/toxin exposure	Long-term use is safe Resveratrol is found in grapes, berries, pistachios, peanuts, and cocoa

Therapy	Mechanism	Dose or activity	Remarks
Capsaicin [55]	NRF2 activator	Best used from food—*Capsicum frutescens* (chilli pepper) 500 mg per day of dried chilli powder in capsule	Dietary sources are plentiful in many chilli pepper products
Berberine [56]	MAPK activator and mitohormetin	Berberine sulphate 500 mg bid Berberine bound to phosphatidyl choline (phytosome) will have better absorption, although the alkaloid is absorbed adequately without being in that form	This has effects on regulating blood sugar as well as the mitohormetic effects Berberine and similar alkaloids are found in *Hydrastis canadensis* *Mahonia* (Berberis) *aquafolia, M. vulgaris* *Coptis chinensis* While generally safe, it is an isoquinoline alkaloid and does require a fully functioning liver to metabolize higher amounts

Therapies to support antioxidant systems

Therapy	Mechanism	Dose	Remarks
Ascorbic acid (vitamin C) [57]	Directly neutralizes free radicals Required for enzyme glutathione reductase Supports levels of superoxide dismutase (SOD)	Varies depending on body mass, diet, and objectives: 500–3000 mg orally I.V. Ascorbic acid per physician prescription (doses may range from 1 g to 10 g)	Some patients report loose stools after taking vitamin C Buffered forms such as calcium ascorbate may be used but should consider the patient needs tolerance of calcium or sodium I.V. Ascorbic acid is used in very high doses as part of an integrative cancer treatment approach
Manganese [31]	Required cofactor for superoxide dismutase (SOD) 2—Active in the mitochondrial matrix	1–8 mg of manganese from amino acid chelate (manganese bisglycinate chelate, manganese glycinate chelate, and manganese aspartate)	Dietary sources should be considered strongly: Whole grains, clams, oysters, mussels, nuts, soybeans and other legumes, rice, leafy vegetables, coffee, tea, and many spices such as black pepper

Therapy	Mechanism	Dose	Remarks
Copper [31]	Required for SOD 1 and SOD 3, which is active in mitochondrial membrane, cytoplasm, extracellular matrix, cell membrane	2000 mcg a day of copper from the forms copper biglycinate or copper citrate Do not give excessive amounts	Not a common deficiency, strongly consider dietary sources: Shellfish, seeds and nuts, organ meats, wheat-bran cereals, whole-grain products, and chocolate Those with higher zinc intakes need more copper
Zinc [31]	Required for SOD 1 and SOD 3, which is active in mitochondrial membrane, cytoplasm, extracellular matrix, cell membrane	15–30 mg of zinc per day as zinc glycinate or zinc picolinate	Can be deficient due to malabsorption of dietary deficiency. Phytates from grains can chelate zinc and decrease bioavailability Food sources are meat, fish, and seafood and to a lesser degree eggs and dairy products Legumes, nuts, and whole grains contain zinc but is less bioavailable

Therapy	Mechanism	Dose	Remarks
Dietary protein, including cysteine, glycine, and glutamic acid [32]	Required for the manufacture of glutathione, which is central to free radical control (including the conversion of H_2O_2 created by SOD to H_2O)	Protein intake should be 0.8 gram per kg body mass S-adenosylmethionine 200 mg per day to promote cysteine formation	SAM-e might also promote methionine production depending on body needs. It is first converted to homocysteine (if not made into cysteine) and adequate methylfolate must be present to convert homocysteine to methionine

References

1. Ewald C. The Matrisome during aging and longevity: a systems-level approach toward defining matreotypes promoting healthy aging. Gerontology. 2019;13:1–9.
2. Statzer C, Park JYC, Ewald CY. Extracellular matrix dynamics as an emerging yet understudied Hallmark of aging and longevity. Aging Dis. 2022;14(3):670–93.
3. Selman M, Pardo A. Fibroageing: an ageing pathological feature driven by dysregulated extracellular matrix-cell mechanobiology. Ageing Res Rev. 2021;70:101393.
4. Levi N, Papismadov N, Solomonov I, Sagi I, Krizhanovsky V. The ECM path of senescence in aging: components and modifiers. FEBS J. 2020;287(13):2636–46.
5. Sun Y, Li W, Lu Z, Chen R, Ling J, Ran Q, et al. Rescuing replication and osteogenesis of aged mesenchymal stem cells by exposure to a young extracellular matrix. FASEB J. 2011;25(5):1474–85.
6. Heinz A. Elastases and elastokines: elastin degradation and its significance in health and disease. Crit Rev Biochem Mol Biol. 2020;55(3):252–73.
7. Thomson J, Singh M, Eckersley A, Cain SA, Sherratt MJ, Baldock C. Fibrillin microfibrils and elastic fibre proteins: functional interactions and extracellular regulation of growth factors. Semin Cell Dev Biol. 2019;89:109–17.

8. Jakimiuk K, Gesek J, Atanasov AG, Tomczyk M. Flavonoids as inhibitors of human neutrophil elastase. J Enzyme Inhib Med Chem. 2021;36(1):1016–28.
9. Demkow U, van Overveld FJ. Role of elastases in the pathogenesis of chronic obstructive pulmonary disease: implications for treatment. Eur J Med Res. 2010;15(S2)
10. Twarda-Clapa A, Olczak A, Białkowska AM, Koziołkiewicz M. Advanced glycation end-products (AGEs): formation, chemistry, classification, receptors, and diseases related to AGEs. Cells. 2022;11(8):1312.
11. Mebratu YA, Soni S, Rosas LE, Rojas M, Horowitz JC, Nho RS. The aged extracellular matrix and the profibrotic role of senescence-associated secretory phenotype. Am J Physiol Cell Physiol. 2023;325(3):C565–79.
12. Wang Z, Walker GW, Muir DCG, Nagatani-Yoshida K. Toward a global understanding of chemical pollution: a first comprehensive analysis of national and regional chemical inventories. Environ Sci Technol. 2020;54(5):2575–84.
13. Park JYC, King A, Björk V, English BW, Fedintsev A, Ewald CY. Strategic outline of interventions targeting extracellular matrix for promoting healthy longevity. Am J Physiol Cell Physiol. 2023;325(1):C90–128.
14. Tang GY, Meng X, Gan RY, Zhao CN, Liu Q, Feng YB, et al. Health functions and related molecular mechanisms of tea components: an update review. Int J Mol Sci. 2019;20(24):6196.
15. Ewald CY. Drug screening implicates chondroitin sulfate as a potential longevity pill. Front Aging. 2021;2
16. Cj B. Metformin: historical overview. Diabetologia. 2017. Available from: https://pubmed.ncbi.nlm.nih.gov/28776081/
17. Horng CT, Wu HC, Chiang NN, Lee CF, Huang YS, Wang HY, et al. Inhibitory effect of burdock leaves on elastase and tyrosinase activity. Exp Ther Med. 2017;14(4):3247–52.
18. Dudek M, Swift J, Meng QJ. The circadian clock and extracellular matrix homeostasis in aging and age-related diseases. Am J Physiol Cell Physiol. 2023;325(1):C52–9.
19. Vasey C, McBride J, Penta K. Circadian rhythm dysregulation and restoration: the role of melatonin. Nutrients. 2021;13(10):3480.
20. Uysal N, Kizildag S, Yuce Z, Guvendi G, Kandis S, Koc B, et al. Timeline (bioavailability) of magnesium compounds in hours: which magnesium compound works best? Biol Trace Elem Res. 2019;187(1):128–36.
21. Kerch G. Role of changes in state of bound water and tissue stiffness in development of age-related diseases. Polymers. 2020;12(6):1362.
22. Choi S, Ham S, Lee YI, Kim J, Lee WJ, Lee JH. Silibinin downregulates types I and III collagen expression via suppression of the mTOR signaling pathway. Int J Mol Sci. 2023;24(18):14386.

23. CDC. FastStats. www.cdc.gov. 2020. Available from: https://www.cdc.gov/nchs/fastats/diet.htm
24. Holwerda AM, van Loon LJC. The impact of collagen protein ingestion on musculoskeletal connective tissue remodeling: a narrative review. Nutr Rev. 2021;80(6):1497.
25. Campos LD, et al. Collagen supplementation in skin and orthopedic diseases: a review of the literature. Heliyon. 2023;9(4):e14961.
26. Singh P, Gollapalli K, Mangiola S, Schranner D, Yusuf MA, Chamoli M, et al. Taurine deficiency as a driver of aging. Science. 2023;380(6649):eabn9257.
27. Kritikaki E, Asterling R, Ward L, Padget K, Barreiro E, C. M. Simoes D. Exercise training-induced extracellular matrix protein adaptation in locomotor muscles: a systematic review. Cells. 2021;10(5):1022.
28. Commonfund. Molecular Transducers of Physical Activity in Humans. commonfund.nih.gov. 2015. Available from: https://commonfund.nih.gov/moleculartransducers
29. Rees MD, Kennett EC, Whitelock JM, Davies MJ. Oxidative damage to extracellular matrix and its role in human pathologies. Free Radic Biol Med. 2008;44(12):1973–2001.
30. Kennett EC, Chuang CY, Degendorfer G, Whitelock JM, Davies MJ. Mechanisms and consequences of oxidative damage to extracellular matrix. Biochem Soc Trans. 2011;39(5):1279–87.
31. Fukai T, Ushio-Fukai M. Superoxide Dismutases: role in redox signaling, vascular function, and diseases. Antioxid Redox Signal. 2011;15(6):1583–606.
32. Minich DM, Brown BI. A review of dietary (Phyto)nutrients for glutathione support. Nutrients. 2019;11(9):2073.
33. Lubos E, Loscalzo J, Handy DE. Glutathione peroxidase-1 in health and disease: from molecular mechanisms to therapeutic opportunities. Antioxid Redox Signal. 2011;15(7):1957–97.
34. Bernhoft RA. Mercury toxicity and treatment: a review of the literature. J Environ Public Health. 2011;2012(460508):1–10.
35. Calabrese EJ. Historical foundations of wound healing and its potential for acceleration: dose-response considerations. Wound Repair Regen. 2013;21(2):180–93.
36. Calabrese EJ, Osakabe N, Di Paola R, Siracusa R, Fusco R, D'Amico R, et al. Hormesis defines the limits of lifespan. Ageing Res Rev. 2023;91:102074.
37. Calabrese E. Hormesis: path and progression to significance. Int J Mol Sci. 2018;19(10):2871.
38. Bárcena C, Mayoral P, Quirós PM. Mitohormesis, an Antiaging Paradigm. Int Rev Cell Mol Biol. 2018;340:35–77.
39. Cheng YW, Liu J, Finkel T. Mitohormesis. Cell Metab. 2023;35(11):1872–86.

40. Tharp KM, Higuchi-Sanabria R, Timblin GA, Ford B, Garzon-Coral C, Schneider C, et al. Adhesion-mediated mechanosignaling forces mitohormesis. Cell Metab. 2021;33(7):1322–41.
41. Thring TS, Hili P, Naughton DP. Anti-collagenase, anti-elastase and antioxidant activities of extracts from 21 plants. BMC Complement Altern Med. 2009;9(1)
42. Wittenauer J, Mäckle S, Sußmann D, Schweiggert-Weisz U, Carle R. Inhibitory effects of polyphenols from grape pomace extract on collagenase and elastase activity. Fitoterapia. 2015;101:179–87.
43. Liu L, Wen T, Xiao Y, Chen H, Yang S, Shen X. Sea buckthorn extract mitigates chronic obstructive pulmonary disease by suppression of ferroptosis via scavenging ROS and blocking p53/MAPK pathways. J Ethnopharmacol. 2025;336:118726.
44. Sławińska N, Żuchowski J, Stochmal A, Olas B. Extract from sea buckthorn seeds – a phytochemical, antioxidant, and hemostasis study; effect of thermal processing on its chemical content and biological activity in vitro. Nutrients. 2023;15(3):686.
45. Bokhari J, Khan MR, Shabbir M, Rashid U, Jan S, Zai JA. Evaluation of diverse antioxidant activities of Galium aparine. Spectrochim Acta A Mol Biomol Spectrosc. 2013;102:24–9.
46. Fhayli W, Boëté Q, Kihal N, Cenizo V, Sommer P, Boyle WA, et al. Dill extract induces elastic fiber Neosynthesis and functional improvement in the ascending aorta of aged mice with reversal of age-dependent cardiac hypertrophy and involvement of Lysyl oxidase-Like-1. Biomol Ther. 2020;10(2):173.
47. Song SY, Lee SH, Bae MS, Park DH, Cho SS. Strong inhibition of xanthine oxidase and elastase of *Baccharis trimera* (less.) DC stem extract and analysis of biologically active constituents. Front Pharmacol. 2023;14:1160330.
48. Babu PVA, Gokulakrishnan A, Dhandayuthabani R, Ameethkhan D, Kumar CVP, Ahamed MIN. Protective effect of Withania somnifera (Solanaceae) on collagen glycation and cross-linking. Comp Biochem Physiol B Biochem Mol Biol. 2007;147(2):308–13.
49. Vidal C, Zhu W, Manohar S, Aydın B, Keiderling TA, Messersmith PB, et al. Collagen-collagen interactions mediated by plant-derived proanthocyanidins: a spectroscopic and atomic force microscopy study. Acta Biomater. 2016;41:110–8.
50. Lee Y, Field JM, Sehgal A. Circadian rhythms, disease and chronotherapy. J Biol Rhythm. 2021;36(6):503–31.
51. Wirz-Justice A, Skene D, Munch M. The relevance of daylight for humans. Biochem Pharmacol. 2020;191:114304.
52. Cheung KL, Kong AN. Molecular targets of dietary Phenethyl Isothiocyanate and Sulforaphane for cancer chemoprevention. AAPS J. 2009;12(1):87–97.

53. Li X, Sun P, Zhang D, Yan L. Curcumin in vitro neuroprotective effects are mediated by p62/keap-1/Nrf2 and PI3K/AKT signaling pathway and autophagy inhibition. Physiol Res. 2023;72:497–510.
54. Qin X, Niu W, Zhao K, Luo Y, Wang W, He Y, et al. Resveratrol enhances post-injury muscle regeneration by regulating antioxidant and mitochondrial biogenesis. Curr Res Food Sci. 2025;10:100972.
55. Varshney V, Kumar A, Parashar V, Kumar A, Goyal A, Garabadu D. Therapeutic potential of capsaicin in various neurodegenerative diseases with special focus on Nrf2 signaling. Curr Pharm Biotechnol. 2024;25(13):1693–707.
56. Han CY, Sun TT, Xv GP, Wang SS, Gu JG, Liu CY. Berberine ameliorates CCl4-induced liver injury in rats through regulation of the Nrf2-Keap1-ARE and p53 signaling pathways. Mol Med Rep. 2019;20(4):3095–102.
57. Gęgotek A, Skrzydlewska E. Ascorbic acid as antioxidant. Vitam Horm. 2023;121:247–70.

7 Disordered Circulation and Communication: Examples of Extracellular Matrix Involvement and Treatment

The extracellular matrix (ECM) is essential to the circulation of nutrients, and gasses among cells and through tissues. It is also integral to communication via the autonomic nervous system. It is also communicatory via the nucleus to cytoskeleton to integrin to matrix protein network. It may also communicate via more extensive fascial connections, which permeate the entire body.

Oxygen, glucose, and nutrients must leave the capillaries and move through the ECM in order to come to the cell membrane. The ECM is naturally a good conduit for these vital substances. But when the ECM is abnormal, this circulation becomes less efficient [1].

The polysaccharide nature of ECM gel allows this diffusion. Water is always bound to the matrix, which lends itself to dispersal of nutrients to the cells, and wastes from the cells to local lymph collection. In more dense tissues, nutrients are diffused to the majority of hyaline and elastic cartilage via the perichondrium surrounding cartilage or the synovial fluid in the case of articular hyaline cartilage. Perichondrium is a dense irregular collagenous protective connective tissue, rich in fibroblasts, chondrogenic cells, and chondroblasts.

Communication within a tissue and the rest of the body can be altered by changes to the ECM. Many cellular growth factors are contained in vesicles within the ECM. Hyaluronic acid can bind these vesicles as can glycoprotein structures. Sudden degradation

F. Smith, *The Extracellular Matrix in Health and Disease*,
https://doi.org/10.1007/978-3-031-94465-9_7

of the ECM can release too many growth factors, causing an imbalance in the local tissue structure.

Mechanotransduction is a type of communication in the ECM where proteins and glycoproteins, by their connection to integrin or CD44 proteins, send mechanical inputs to the cell microstructure, which ultimately connects to the cell nucleus [2]. This can influence cellular genetic expression. Mechanotranduction has both nuclear and mitochondrial effects. Embryogenesis, as well as healing from injury, involves intricate mechanosensing and genomic response sequences.

The fascial system is a living network of proteins and the fibroblasts throughout the body at both superficial and deep levels of tissue [3]. It is connected to the extracellular matrix of surrounding structures and fascial layers themselves are imbued with extracellular matrix. The fascia is also richly innervated. It can cycle through stages of contraction and relaxation throughout the day. Through a phenomenon known as biotensegrity, the structural rearrangements of fascia support massive amounts of stress, and changes in one locality (such as contracting around an injured local tissue) are felt by fascial components elsewhere.

Factors that can interfere with normal circulation and coordination in the extracellular matrix are the following.

Fibrosis

Crosslinked collagen is a normal finding in the ECM. With aging, as seen in the discussion on hypofunction, crosslinking becomes more permanent, and tissues become stiffer (which is also due to the eventual wearing out of elastin) [4]. But one abnormal situation is that of massive collagen deposition due to fibrosis. This can be a true scar due to healing by second intention. But often the deposition of large amounts of collagen, which can become crosslinked enzymatically and nonenzymatically, is a response to chronic injury (Fig. 7.1). The advent of cirrhosis in a chronically inflamed liver is a classic example. But most tissues and all organs exhibit this phenomenon. When fibrosis occurs, the physical transit of lymph, nutrients, various solutes, chemical messengers, and immune cells through the ECM is interrupted.

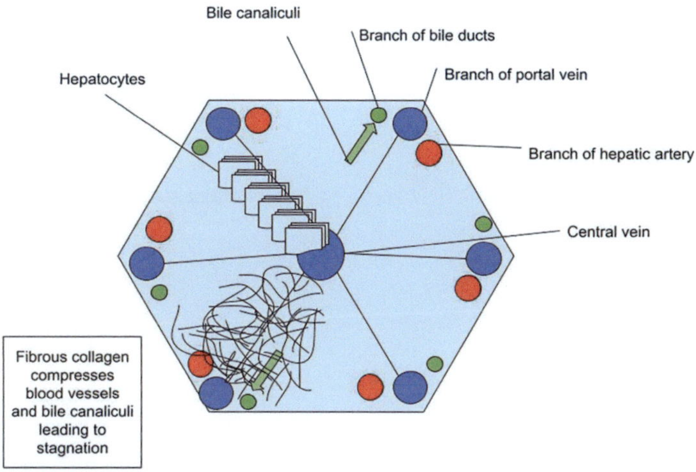

Fig. 7.1 Fibrosis and hepatic triad

Edema

Edema is the trapping of fluid in the interstitium and eventually infiltrates into fascial planes. It can be caused by excessive leakage of blood vessels or stagnation of local venous channels. Inflammation will automatically cause some edema, mediated by histamine, bradykinin, and other messengers. Another cause can be dysfunction within the ECM itself. Integrin seems to have an effect on the signals that lead to fluid flow. It is important to remember that the ECM will naturally, and beneficially, trap large amounts of water. Hyaluronic acid and glycosaminoglycans in general act as water traps. This creates a hydrated colloid in the ECM. That leads to better biochemical function as well as a structural fullness that is noticeable when it is disturbed.

Edema will itself begin to injure the ECM [5]. The stagnation that occurs leads to the accumulation of metabolic toxins in the area. This can degrade the health of tissues. Fluid and lymph expungement is part of the normal maintenance of tissues. This event occurs in the central nervous system via the glymphatic system (Fig. 7.2), mostly at night. So, when the circulation of lymph in the ECM is lacking, the ECM is already on its way to having

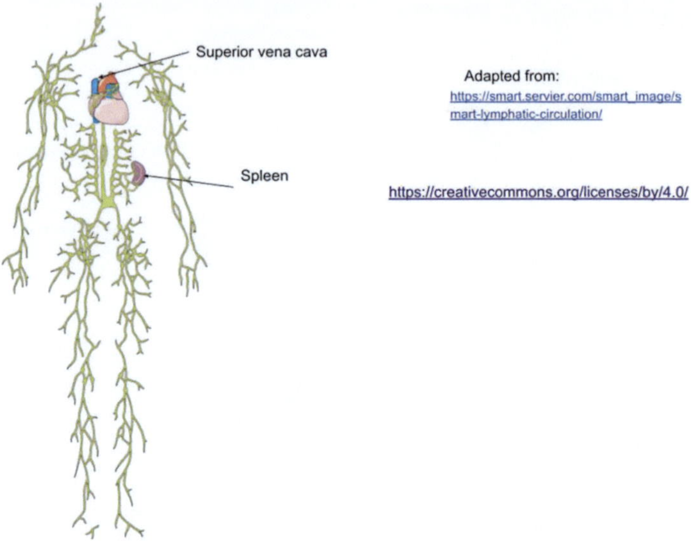

Fig. 7.2 Lymphatic system

damage to its proteins, glycoproteins, proteoglycans, and various microstructures.

Inflammation

This is the topic of upcoming chapters, but in terms of flow and communication, inflammation leads to excessive fluid accumulation and a certain amount of fibrin-producing activity. This is why post injury, athletic training and physical therapies will work to mobilize and massage injured tissues, to reduce strictures/adhesions and help with the healthy inflow of blood and nutrients, and outflow of carbon dioxide, lactate, and other metabolic toxins. It has to be remembered that cells are only in proximity to microvessels of the circulatory system, all nutrients must pass through the ECM, and all cellular wastes must also do so.

Insulin Dysregulation

Hyperinsulinemia can be exacerbated or caused by changes to the ECM [6, 7]. Excessive deposits of collagen and fibrillar proteins in general can have a blocking effect on insulin, preventing it from reaching the cell. The alternation of ECM to become stiffer due to the accumulation of advanced glycation end products (AGE) can also block insulin from the cell. The type of, or excessive of, the transmembrane protein integrin in muscle cells can also lead to insulin resistance. This can occur under conditions of chronic inflammation, which will also impair matrix metalloproteinase activity, leading to more protein accumulation and increased matrix stiffness. The space from capillary endothelium to cell membrane becomes harder to traverse for insulin. Moreover, under these inflammatory conditions, certain types of integrin that have an alpha subunit begin to predominate. These integrin formations lead to a suppression of GLUT4 migration to the muscle cell membrane. This seems to be mediated by a change in cellular tyrosine kinase activity. Thus, insulin, which can arrive at the insulin receptor, will be less effective in increasing GLUT4 activity, and thus there is less glucose transport into the muscle cells. Similar effects are found in the liver itself, leading to more hepatic glucose formation, and in adipose tissue, leading to less ability of adipocytes to absorb glucose.

Dysfunction of the Glymphatic System

Brain ECM lacks collagen and fibrillar proteins and is good at rapid absorption and discharge of water—a high-functioning endothelial glycocalyx is important for CSF drainage. The brain extracellular matrix is very low in collagen and fibrillar proteins, and very high in hyaluronic acid. This makes the brain very good at holding water, and it can take in, and under the right conditions, discharge fluids, very quickly. The interstitial fluid of the brain is the cerebral spinal fluid and circulates through ventricles. Not all substances can find their way into the brain, tight endothelial junctions that sit across from astrocyte endfeet create a so-called blood–brain barrier. The choroid plexus cells produce the CSF. The choroid cells have various transport proteins and have much control over what molecules are granted entry into the brain. Unlike the rest of the body, lymph cannot just drain into pericapillary areas and directly into the lymphatics. A special drainage system where the toxins such as beta-amyloid and synuclein are discharged exists and is called the "glymphatic system" (Fig. 7.3). This flushing of CFS into the venous system takes place as toxins in the extracellular matrix of the brain are washed out by the astrocytic endfeet (which surround the brain vasculature), which have a water secreting transmembrane protein called aquaporin-4 (AQP4).

Improper glymphatic flow has been found in rodent models, and in human studies, to be associated with less discharge of beta-amyloid, which is found in various types of dementia and is a

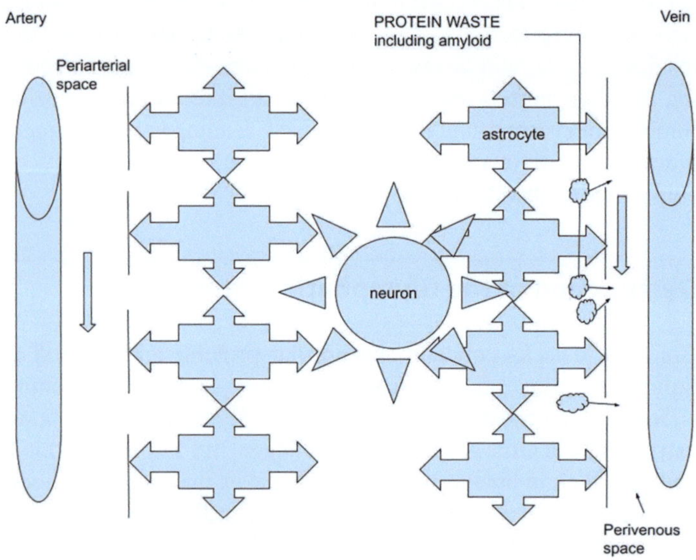

Fig. 7.3 Glymphatic system

contributor to neurodegeneration. This discharge does not happen unless the brain and the body are in a state of deep relaxation, and this mainly occurs in the deeper levels of sleep, particularly during slow-wave sleep, which the American Academy of Sleep Medicine terms stage 3 sleep [8].

Dysregulation of Circadian Rhythms

The body has central and peripheral clocks, with central pathways set by the suprachiasmatic nuclei of the hypothalamus. That brain region is informed by light stimulation to the retina. Tissues and organs have their own "zeitgebers," which synchronize to the central clock. Circadian dysregulation due to sleep issues, travel across time zones, lack of sunlight including winter in higher latitudes, and shift work is well known. Aging dysregulates the circadian rhythms, and even though the basic genetic requirements for a normal circadian activity (such as the CLOCK gene) remain, the transcription of and transport of necessary proteins are impaired. This is hastened by too much sirtuin activation (as a result of mitochondrial stress) and over-activation of mTOR.

Changes and dysregulation of circadian rhythms in a tissue will impact the local extracellular matrix [9]. This can impact matrix metalloproteinase activity, vesicles that contain cell signaling molecules, and collagen secretion. The ECM can change during aging and can affect the local zeitgebers. For example, fibroblasts have a circadian rhythm and impacts their secretory function. The release of matrix metalloproteinases by macrophages in the matrix follows a circadian cycle as well (Fig. 7.4). The disruption of circadian rhythms can disturb the ECM, but matrix changes also impact the circadian rhythms. A softer, more pliable ECM supports circadian function, and a stiffer matrix will impair normal circadian functioning in tissues at a local level. This effect appears to be transmitted to the nucleus via the cytoskeleton, like many force-sensing effects of the cell and ECM interaction.

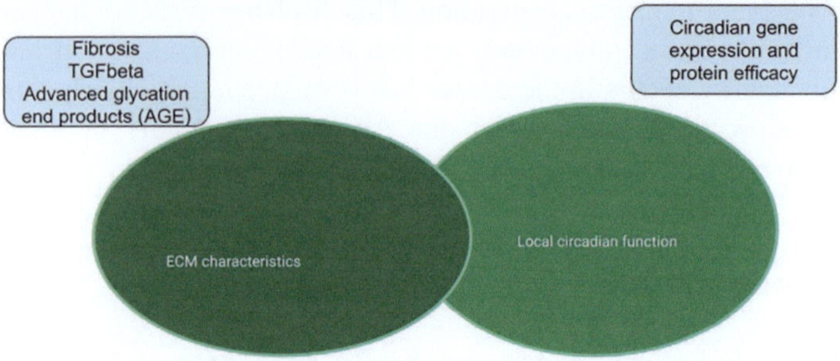

Fig. 7.4 Circadian rhythms

Treatments That Encourage Matrix Regulation and Lymph Drainage

Diet

Spermidine is a polyamine found in the human body and many organisms. It is a naturally produced inducer of autophagy and levels can decrease during aging [10]. Spermidine can decrease inflammation in lymphatic vessels [11]. It can be taken as a supplement (see below) and is also found in foods. These foods include durian fruit, shiitake mushrooms, fresh green pepper, wheat germ, amaranth grain, cauliflower, and broccoli. It is also found in fermented foods, including natto and naturally aged cheeses. Bonetti et al. and Jeong et al. report that spermidine decreases TNF-α, IL-1β, NO, and PGE2.

An anti-inflammatory diet that helps regulate insulin and blood sugar diets is important for reducing lymphatic inflammation [12]. The diabetogenic aspects of contemporary diets in developed countries and beyond have excessively refined carbohydrate sources, as well as chemically extracted vegetable oils that have a disproportionate amount of free radical-propagating compounds in them relative to natural antioxidants such as tocopherols, carotenoids, and phenolics.

Polyphenols in general are helpful to prevent the inflammation and fibrin deposition in lymph stagnation. Plant-derived coumarins are also helpful, in that they enhance localized circulation [12, 13].

Although sodium is an essential nutrient, patients who show signs of poor lymph flow should limit salt intake. Sodium can have a fluid-retaining effect, which can exacerbate localized stagnation [14]. The increased hydrostatic pressure due to excessive sodium intake can drive lymphedema. Excessive phytoestrogens might contribute to this via an estrogen effect, but this does not mean that phytoestrogens (legumes and other foods) need to be avoided, but might need to be limited, especially soy (*Glycine max*). By the same token, excessive xenoestrogens can lead to edema and fluid retention via estrogenic effects. In a dietary sense, this means that storing and cooking food in plastic is to be avoided. Likewise, food prepared on plastic cutting boards, rice not washed before cooking (washed rice is better), so-called "Himalayan salt" (which is from the salt range mountains in Pakistan), and water from plastic bottles need to be limited or avoided.

Dietary Supplements

The extracts of olive, *Olea europa*, contain hydroxytyrosol, a phenolic compound. It has anti-inflammatory properties that specifically benefits inflamed lymphatic vessels.

Dietary supplements contain hydroxytyrosol as well as spermidine, hesperidin, and vitamin A. Hesperidin is a well-known citrus bioflavonoid that decreases vascular permeability. Pryznska has outlined the many biological activities of hesperidin in a 2022 review, and it has strong anti-inflammatory activities in the circulatory system [15]. Vitamin A is anti-inflammatory and has a metabolite, retinoic acid, which may help some lymphedema patients who have a mutation in a gene known as RORC.

Hormetic Inputs

Hormesis is the use of very low-dose stimulation to create a counter-response from the body. Hormetins can often lead to an adaptation that is positive. Professor Edward Calabrese outlined the principles of hormesis in the 1990s, and extensive research, refinement, and applications of hormetic studies have occurred since then [16].

Biological medicine is a type of therapy that originated in Europe. It overlaps with homeopathy, although many biological therapies are in the low-dose zone for herbs and minerals. One example of a biological medicine that can impact lymph draining is Lymphomyosot (Biologische Heilmittel Heel GmbH, Baden-Baden, Germany), a medicine that contains diluted herbal extracts and minerals [17].

One ampoule (containing fluid for the injection of 1 mL of Lymphomyosot) contains 0.55 mg *Gentiana lutea* D5, 0.55 mg *Pinus sylvestris* D4, 0.55 mg *Scrophularia nodosa* D3, 0.55 mg *Equisetum hiemale* D4, 1.1 mg *Ferrum jodatum* D12, 0.55 mg *Calcium phosphoricum* D12, 0.55 mg *Aranea diadematus* D6, 0.55 mg *Fumaria officinalis* D4, 1.1 mg *Geranium robertianum* D4, 0.55 mg *Levothyroxinum* D12, 1.1 mg *Nasturtium officinale* D4, 0.55 mg *Natrium sulfuricum* D4, 0.55 mg *Sarsaparillae radix* D6, 0.55 mg *Myosotis arvensis* D3, 0.55 mg *Teucrium scorodonia* D3, 0.55 mg *Veronica officinalis* D3, sodium chloride, and water. All components are prepared according to the European Pharmacopoeia. Lymphomyosot has decreased edema in experimental models. The "D" next to these substances refers to 1 in 10 dilutions. A D3 means that a tincture of the substance has been serially diluted three times.

Manual Therapies

There are various manual therapies to increase lymph flow. The general principle is mobilization of lymph, and drainage toward the central part of the body. Lymph normally moves toward the lymphatic duct, which empties into the right and left subclavian veins (named the right lymphatic duct and on the left side of the thorax, named the thoracic duct).

In order to get congested lymph to start to flow, the initial part of a manual approach is a gentle lifting and rolling of the skin, centripetally, toward the center of the body. This is done on the limbs and can also be done on the lower back, abdomen, and upper back and posterior neck. This is followed up by deeper and slower stroking movements of the hands on the limbs to push lymph along to the center of the body [18–20].

Electrical therapies are a possibility for lymph stagnation. These gentle electrical current therapies can create local (smaller areas of tissues including their ECM) and more systemic (flow of the lymph system across larger body regions) effects.

Electrical therapies can involve DC (direct) current, which has been the most studied in cellular and animal models. Electrical current seems to open up voltage-gated channels, leading to relaxation of tissues, and it has a lymphangiogenesis, that is, it causes an increase in the number of lymph vessels via release of trophic factors. It leads to decreased fibrin and inflammation and also leads to better protein drainage from an area. There are wound-healing aspects to electrical current, which is important in later-stage lymphedema where localized inflammation is destroying tissues. The more ECM-specific microdrainage of the interstitium is of interest in that this is an area that is aided by manual therapy but not as directly impacted by it. Electrical therapies can work at a very small, local level.

In a study comparing low-intensity electrical therapy with manual therapy for breast cancer-related lymphedema, the electrical stimulation was not superior in drainage but decreased pain and improved quality of life. Perhaps the localized effects allowed for better cellular metabolic waste disposal, and regionally, there is still improvement (if not superior to manual decongestion therapy) of lymph out of affected regions [21].

Hydrotherapy

Hydrotherapy is a blanket term for treatments involving the application of water to the human body. This almost always involves a deliberate selection of

(a) Water temperature.
(b) Consistency and alternations of temperatures.

(c) Durations of treatment or phases of treatment of different temperature.
(d) Delivery form (immersion, sheets or towels soaked in water, steam, etc.)

For example, a patient might be given a 5-min application of warm towels to the abdomen, followed by application of towels wrung out in cold water to the same area, which are left in place until they reach a temperature similar to the test of the body surface. This action initially enhances circulation to the area by a vasodilation effect. Unlike passively soaking in hot water, as in a hot tub, this initial vasodilation is followed by a cold exposure to the area. While this is initially vasoconstrictive, provided that the cold exposure is transient (and not overwhelming such as repeated ice packs), the body will respond by diverting more circulation to the area in order to establish a more regular temperature. This is a homeostatic response that is mediated by the autonomic nervous system as well as the hypothalamus.

The use of physical agents such as water of differing temperatures can modulate the flow of blood and lymph to, and from a tissue. This has a decongestant effect in the way that it can better drain metabolic wastes from the area. It has a nourishing effect in that it can bring oxygen and nutrients to tissues.

This alone provides more opportunities for the exchange of nutrients, gasses, and toxins in and out of the ECM. But there appear to be some direct ECM effects of hydrotherapy [22].

Sleep Quality and the Glymphatic System

This is of utmost importance for impaired glymphatic circulation, which can eventually lead to amyloid accumulation in the brain. The activation of AQP4 channels to drain CSF required slow-wave brain activity as well as relaxation of the vascular system itself [23].

Magnesium can be helpful for sleep issues. A significant portion of the population is magnesium deficient. A 2023 systematic review found that magnesium status was associated with sleep quality, but magnesium supplementation did not show a strong association with sleep improvement. Although this area needs more investigation given the widespread nature of magnesium deficiency, it points to the fact that those who lack magnesium will have improved sleep when their levels are normalized. Those who have adequate or even good magnesium levels might not find that sleep problems are improved—as those problems are probably due to other issues such as stress, pain, circadian rhythms, and apnea. That being said, there are randomized controlled trials that show improvements in mental alertness and sleep quality with magnesium supplementation, and it remains a strong consideration for naturopathic treatments to address sleep quality [24].

Magnesium can be dosed at an additional 500 mg per day, although some studies go higher. The issue with magnesium is that absorption is limited, and unabsorbed magnesium will lead to osmotic diarrhea and abdominal cramping. Magnesium malate appears to have better absorption, including studies that measure red blood cell magnesium levels over time. A study by Weiss et al. (2018) found significant improvements in red blood cell magnesium in a deficient population using a dimagnesium malate supplement, which was well tolerated.

Magnesium serum concentrations are more likely to fluctuate and the RBC assay is a better test. Only 0.3% of total body magnesium is found in serum. Serum concentrations can be a screening test with valid uses for uncovering deficiency and indicating rapid changes of status. Magnesium citrate or even oxide, or amino acid chelated magnesium, does provide the ion, but the malate form appears to be most effective in getting from intestinal lumen into the circulation.

Vitamin B12 is sometimes helpful for sleep, certainly in those with low cobalamin levels. There is also an association between low levels of B12 and narcolepsy. Supplementation in the diet through B12, in foods of animal origin, will easily provide the RDA of 2.4 mcg for adults. However, some individuals will have absorption issues or have dietary patterns that exclude B12. If the absorption issues are the cause, then sublingual B12 (which tends to come in doses of 1000 mcg per drop) or B12 intramuscular injection can treat it.

Glymphatic drainage appears to be encouraged by exercise, alcohol restriction, and not only enough quality sleep, but sleep position. A right-sided sleep position, and not too many hours spent supine, encourages glymphatic drainage. Patients have difficulty tracking this on their own; a sleep lab or perhaps diligent self-recording is the best way to know what sleep position is.

Sleep Supporting Botanical Medicines

Valeriana officinalis (Valerian) is a traditional sleep aid and nervine. It acts on the GABA (gamma amino butyric acid) system of the nervous system, which has an inhibitory effect. The compounds from Valerian, such as valepotriates and valerenic acid, act to reduce anxiety and relax muscles. Both of these effects are helpful in sleep. Musculoskeletal relaxation is an early part of the sleep cycle, but so is mental calmness. Valerian does not work for everyone, but in sleep clinical trials, it has shown itself to be quite effective. It does not typically create any morning grogginess. Because it is a mild sedative, any patient who has a history of addiction should use it with supervision and with some caution, especially if sedative drugs were part of their problem.

A 2020 Systematic Review of 60 studies involving Valerian and sleep found benefits, but much inconsistency between delivery forms of Valerian (preparations made from root/rhizome are more potent) and product quality (which can be uneven in the dietary supplement market). This underscores the importance of a high-quality preparation made from either a water and ethanol extract (for those who are able to consume this small amount of ethanol daily) to standardized extracts, which range from 0.8% to 2.0% valerenic acid. Many herbal medicines, including *Valeriana officinalis*, have a range of compounds that have affinity for multiple targets. Therefore, standardization of one single compound can be used as a quality indicator, but is not the sole criterion for the medicine's effectiveness [25].

Fascial Mobilization and Realignment

The fascial pathways through the body run across major muscle groups, often with a rotational or twisting pathway. Fascia can be both superficial or deep and is always contiguous with the ECM. This system ought to be flexible and capable of stretch in multiple directions. But the fascia can become stiff, rigid, and contracted. This is partly due to increased collagen and decreased elastin in the ECM. In the conventional medicine setting, myofascial release is somewhat supported by studies that show it can help with low back pain or regional tight muscles. This is found to be somewhat helpful in reducing limitations of function.

In a naturopathic approach, the rehabilitation of the fascial network takes on much more importance. This goes beyond treating an isolated source of pain. Facial networks can become tightened or restricted in the long term, and this can restrict movement. Moreover, the proximity to and connections with the local extracellular matrix mean that fluid flow and nutrient in waste-out circulation of tissues are impacted by fascial flexibility and stability.

Since lymph is extremely connected to fascia and the ECM. Therapies that can release this area such as counterstrain [26], structural integration, or Rolfing [27] and yoga [28] can be helpful. The more widely used decongestant physical therapies continue to be valuable as well [29].

Additional Lymph and Fascia-Supporting Herbs

Plant extracts that support ECM, venous, and lymph tissue are useful for those who have early aging or rapid degeneration of these key components of the lymphatic system. *Astragalus membranaceous* [30] and very small doses of *Artemisia absinthium* [31] (wormwood—a low-dose herb that is contraindicated in pregnancy) can reduce fibrotic reactions. Horse chestnut (*Aesculus hippocastanum*) [13] extract can improve the integrity of vein and collagen tissues in general, as can *Centella asiatica* [13].

Fascia-supporting therapy

Therapy	Mechanism	Application	Remarks
Yoga [28, 32]	Done properly can gently stretch muscles and fascia, and change nervous system tone	With proper instruction, yoga session (45–60 min) twice per week	Yoga can become a regular practice, but for those who engage in other kinds of exercise and meditation, even 2 sessions per week can restore mobility to stiff fascia
Myofascial release exercises [33, 34]	Mechanically stretches fascia and helps condition the fascia to maintain a lower tone; improves elasticity and fascial glide	Done for 10 minutes at least every other day	Foam rollers can be incorporated into myofascial release—Can be taught by practitioners Can be provided by therapist (best) but some efficacy of self/home fascial stretching and release
Fascial counterstrain [26]	Contractions and release of tender, congested, densified, and inflammation areas of fascia	Depend on case, but maybe have weekly visits, or more frequent	Should be performed by practitioners trained in this method Lawrence Jones, DO developed counterstrain in the 1950s and this has been refined and improved by Dr. Brian Tuckey in recent times
Rolfing/ structural integration [27]	Manual stimulation of fascia at a deep level and in selected points	Once a week for 10 sessions, or more	Provided by a practitioner certified in Rolfing or structural integration

Therapy	Mechanism	Application	Remarks
Hydration [35]	In order for fascia to hydrate, expand, de-densify, and glide it needs to be hydrated	Adequate water consumption daily	Although common knowledge, the avoidance of water, use of soft drinks, use of diuretics, and diminished thirst mechanisms with age can lead to various states of dehydration

Anti-inflammatory, antifibrotic therapies

Therapy	Mechanism	Application	Remarks
Artemisia annua (Chinese wormwood) [31]	Antifibrotic mechanisms of artemisinin Prevent the transition of fibroblasts into myofibroblasts	2 ml of tincture (hydroethanol extract) per day 500 mg dried *Artemisia annua* per day	This herb contains thujone, which can be toxic in higher doses. The *A. annua* species has lower thujone content than other forms (such as *Artemisia absinthium*—Wormwood) Contraindicated in pregnancy
Astragalus membranaceus [30]	Antifibrotic properties	5 ml of tincture (hydrothethanol extract) per day 1000 mg of dried *Astragalus membranaceus* per day	Also has immune support and anti-fatigue properties, may be especially useful for those with fibromyalgia and chronic fatigue
Boswellia serrata (Indian frankincense) [36]	Anti-inflammatory to fascia and muscles	400 mg of standardized extract, two times per day	Higher amounts are possible but not always necessary

Physical therapies to increase lymph flow

Therapy	Mechanism	Application	Remarks
Manual therapies [18]	Moves fluid through tissues and encourages flow—Causes reflex activity in the area getting worked on	Various techniques, including effleurage done in centripetal (toward center of body) bodywork In many cases of acute lymphedema, the massaging actions can be more superficial to address trapped fluid, but deeper work can be done A whole-body approach is best.	For regions with acute lymphedema, rule out a localized blood clot (thrombosis) in a vein, before doing any kind of massage
Electrical therapies [21]	Encourages the opening of lymph and venous passages by a depolarizing effect on autonomic local nerves	Provided in office, or, various home devices are on the market	Consider contraindications to this therapy carefully: Pacemaker, electrical instability of heart, pregnancy, etc
Low-dose botanical drainage therapy—such as Lymphomyosot [17]	A low-dose stimulus that encourages a counter-reaction of lymph flow	For low-dose preparations such as Lymphomyosot 10 drops twice a day; 1 tablet twice a day	Also consider traditional botanical lymphatic movers such as *Gallium aperine* (cleavers), the mechanisms of these herbs are still unclear, although there is long traditional use

Therapy	Mechanism	Application	Remarks
Contrast hydrotherapy [22] [37]	Brief warm applications encourage vasodilation, longer cold applications lead to an initial constriction of blood and lymph followed by a reflex increase	Constitutional hydrotherapy with alternating hot and cold applications; local alternating wraps or immersions (i.e., foot bath, or towel wrap to arm)	These can be done as home treatments or in office constitutional hydrotherapy treatments that last about 1 h

Sleep and circadian rhythm support

Therapy	Mechanism	Application	Remarks
Magnesium malate [24]	Regulation of nervous system and muscle tone	300 mg two times per day	Magnesium malate is a well-absorbed form but doses should be separate in order to avoid osmotic diarrhea Other forms of magnesium include citrate, picolinate, gluconate, and (not recommended) oxide
Melatonin [38]	Helps reset circadian rhythm central clock	1 mg 1× per day in the evening Can use higher doses such as 5 mg 1× per day, but starting with less is recommended	Daylight (does not have to be direct sunlight) exposure and limiting artificial sources of light are still important Some foods have melatonin: Cherries, goji berries, pistachios, almonds, milk, and fish

Therapy	Mechanism	Application	Remarks
Valeriana officinalis (valerian) [25]	Compounds such as valerianic acid bind to GABA (gamma amino butyric acid) receptors having a relaxing effect	3 ml 2× per day 5 ml 1× per day before bed Of ethanol-water extract 500 mg of dried valerian in capsules 1× per day or 2× per day	Can use closer to bedtime in order to avoid daytime sedation

References

1. Alberts B, Johnson A, Lewis J, Raff M, Roberts K, Walter P. The extracellular matrix of animals. In: Molecular biology of the cell. 4th ed; 2002. Available from: https://www.ncbi.nlm.nih.gov/books/NBK26810/.
2. Berdiaki A, Neagu M, Tzanakakis P, Spyridaki I, Pérez S, Nikitovic D. Extracellular matrix components and Mechanosensing pathways in health and disease. Biomol Ther. 2024;14(9):1186.
3. Slater AM, Barclay SJ, et al. Fascia as a regulatory system in health and disease. Front Neurol. 2024;15
4. Selman M, Pardo A. Fibroageing: an ageing pathological feature driven by dysregulated extracellular matrix-cell mechanobiology. Ageing Res Rev. 2021;70:101393.
5. Wiig H, Keskin D, Kalluri R. Interaction between the extracellular matrix and lymphatics: consequences for lymphangiogenesis and lymphatic function. Matrix Biol. 2010;29(8):645–56.
6. Ahmad K, Choi I, Lee YH. Implications of skeletal muscle extracellular matrix remodeling in metabolic disorders: diabetes perspective. Int J Mol Sci. 2020;21(11):3845.
7. Williams AS, Kang L, Wasserman DH. The extracellular matrix and insulin resistance. Trends Endocrinol Metab. 2015;26(7):357–66.
8. Hablitz LM, Plá V, Giannetto M, Vinitsky HS, Stæger FF, Metcalfe T, et al. Circadian control of brain glymphatic and lymphatic fluid flow. Nat Commun. 2020;11(1):4411.
9. Williams JM, Yang N, Wood A, Zindy E, Meng QJ, Streuli CH. Epithelial and stromal circadian clocks are inversely regulated by their mechano-matrix environment. J Cell Sci. 2018;131(5)
10. Madeo F, Bauer MA, Carmona-Gutierrez D, Kroemer G. Spermidine: a physiological autophagy inducer acting as an anti-aging vitamin in humans? Autophagy. 2018;15(1):165–8.

11. Karacay C, Prietl B, Harer C, Ehall B, Haudum CW, Bounab K, et al. The effect of spermidine on autoimmunity and beta cell function in NOD mice. Sci Rep. 2022;12(1):4502.
12. Russo B, Picconi F, Malandrucco I, Frontoni S. Flavonoids and insulin-resistance: from molecular evidences to clinical trials. Int J Mol Sci. 2019;20(9)
13. Poage EG, Rodrick JR, Wanchai A, Stewart BR, Cormier JN, Armer JM. Exploring the usefulness of botanicals as an adjunctive treatment for lymphedema: a systematic search and review. PM&R. 2014;7(3):296–310.
14. Goh KP. Management of Hyponatremia. Am Fam Physician. 2004;69(10):2387–94.
15. Pyrzynska K. Hesperidin: a review on extraction methods, stability and biological activities. Nutrients. 2022;14(12):2387.
16. Calabrese EJ. Historical foundations of wound healing and its potential for acceleration: dose-response considerations. Wound Repair Regen. 2013;21(2):180–93.
17. Keim AP, Slis JR, Mendez U, Stroup EM, Burmeister Y, Tsolaki N, et al. The multicomponent medication Lymphomyosot improves the outcome of experimental lymphedema. Lymphat Res Biol. 2013;11(2):81–92.
18. Donahue PMC, Crescenzi R, Petersen KJ, Garza M, Patel N, Lee C, et al. Physical therapy in women with early stage lipedema: potential impact of multimodal manual therapy, compression, exercise, and education interventions. Lymphat Res Biol. 2022;20(4):382–90.
19. Tzani I, Tsichlaki M, Zerva E, Papathanasiou G, Dimakakos E. Physiotherapeutic rehabilitation of lymphedema: state-of-the-art. Lymphology. 2018;51(1):1–12.
20. Brix B, Apich G, Rössler A, Walbrodt S, Goswami N. Effects of physical therapy on hyaluronan clearance and volume regulating hormones in lower limb lymphedema patients: a pilot study. Sci Prog. 2021;104(1):003685042199848.
21. Belmonte R, Tejero M, Ferrer M, Muniesa JM, Duarte E, Cunillera O, et al. Efficacy of low-frequency low-intensity electrotherapy in the treatment of breast cancer-related lymphoedema: a cross-over randomized trial. Clin Rehabil. 2011;26(7):607–18.
22. Mooventhan A, Nivethitha L. Scientific evidence-based effects of hydrotherapy on various Systems of the Body. N Am J Med Sci. 2014;6(5):199.
23. Rasmussen MK, Mestre H, Nedergaard M. Fluid transport in the brain. Physiol Rev. 2022;102(2):1025–151.
24. Arab A, Rafie N, Amani R, Shirani F. The role of magnesium in sleep health: a systematic review of available literature. Biol Trace Elem Res. 2022;201(1):121.
25. Shinjyo N, Waddell G, Green J. Valerian root in treating sleep problems and associated disorders – a systematic review and meta-analysis. Journal of evidence-based. Integr Med. 2020;25(25):2515690X2096732.

26. Fritz K, Novotny K, Carr Jr CL. Physiology, Counterstrain/FPR. PubMed. Treasure Island (FL): StatPearls Publishing; 2021.
27. deLeeuw A. Rolfing therapy: Technique, benefits, and more. Medicalnewstoday.com. Medical News Today; 2022. Available from: https://www.medicalnewstoday.com/articles/rolfing#definition
28. Freguia S, Platano D, Donati D, Giorgi F, Tedeschi R. Closing the gaps: an integrative review of yoga's benefits for lymphedema in breast cancer survivors. Life. 2024;14(8):999.
29. Senger JLB, Kadle RL, Skoracki RJ. Current concepts in the Management of Primary Lymphedema. Medicina. 2023;59(5):894.
30. Liang Y, Chen B, Liang D, Quan XX, Gu R, Zhang M, et al. Pharmacological effects of Astragaloside IV: a review. Molecules. 2023;28(16):6118.
31. Dolivo D, Weathers P, Dominko T. Artemisinin and artemisinin derivatives as anti-fibrotic therapeutics. Acta Pharm Sin B. 2021;11(2):322–39.
32. Little T. A yoga sequence to keep you healthy this winter. Yoga J. 2015;
33. Ajimsha MS, Al-Mudahka NR, Al-Madzhar JA. Effectiveness of myofascial release: systematic review of randomized controlled trials. J Bodyw Mov Ther. 2015;19(1):102–12.
34. Beardsley C, Škarabot J. Effects of self-myofascial release: a systematic review. J Bodyw Mov Ther. 2015;19(4):747–58.
35. Jéquier E, Constant F. Water as an essential nutrient: the physiological basis of hydration. Eur J Clin Nutr. 2019;64(2):115–23.
36. Siddiqui MZ. Boswellia Serrata, a potential Antiinflammatory agent: an overview. Indian J Pharm Sci. 2011;73(3):255–61.
37. Shadgan B, Pakravan AH, Hoens A, Reid WD. Contrast baths, intramuscular hemodynamics, and oxygenation as monitored by near-infrared spectroscopy. J Athl Train. 2018;53(8):782–7.
38. Vasey C, McBride J, Penta K. Circadian rhythm dysregulation and restoration: the role of melatonin. Nutrients. 2021;13(10):3480.

8 Early Inflammation: Examples of Extracellular Matrix Involvement and Treatment

Inflammation is a normal response to injury and part of the body's defense against pathogens [1, 2]. The extracellular matrix is the major theatre of inflammatory events, being an immunologically active zone between cells proper and the vascular endothelium [3]. Inflammation that erupts will usually do some damage to the extracellular matrix, but as inflammation retreats, a phase of resolution can repair the ECM. We can make a distinction between early or acute inflammation and persistent-chronic inflammation. Acute inflammation can be so exuberant that the damage it creates becomes difficult to repair. The ECM may not rebuild itself properly. Recurring damage itself can create more inflammation, a theme of the following chapter. In this chapter, we will examine strategies for regulating inflammation and protecting the ECM, and the cells that live within it.

Inflammation is a normal process in the body and a necessary component of self defense and tissue remodeling [3]. The extracellular matrix has many inflammatory events, which arise from its central role between all cells, and the fact that macrophages and neutrophils are very present in the ECM. One of the normal, low-intensity types of remodeling activity carried about by macrophages is the secretion of matrix metalloproteinases. These enzymes cleave the proteins of the ECM, including collagen. They are kept in check by an inhibitory enzyme—tissue inhibitor of metalloproteinase (TIMPs). There are additional enzymes that

F. Smith, *The Extracellular Matrix in Health and Disease*,
https://doi.org/10.1007/978-3-031-94465-9_8

can cleave matrix proteins, including a family of transmembrane proteins known as a disintegrin and metalloproteinase or ADAM. There is also cathepsin K, from a family of enzymes that mostly operate within lysosomes but can be found in the matrix. There are hyaluronidases that are important maintenance enzymes since so much of the ECM is hyaluronic acid. Elastases are made by neutrophils.

These enzymes, and others, are part of the housekeeping of the ECM, which is a dynamic tissue structure. Their activity does not in itself denote inflammation. But under inflammatory conditions, their activity changes, and they can become part of a purposeful destruction of ECM with a clear resolution in the end or an ongoing destructive process that can in some cases self-perpetuate and propagate.

Inflammation can be triggered by an intrusion or assault by a microorganism, or by trauma. When bacteria enter the ECM, a number of immediate actions of innate immunity occur. The effectors for these responses include phagocytic cells, natural killer cells, the complement system, and the various physical barriers to infection, such as the mucus membranes and skin.

Not only are phagocytic cells such as macrophages and more fixed-in-place Kupffer cells important here, but the antigen processing (as are macrophages) dendritic cells. Also found in the front line of tissues, histiocytes, Kupffer cells, and mast cells are key in initiating inflammation. This is done through the release of histamine, prostaglandins, leukotrienes, oxygen- and nitrogen-derived free radicals, and serotonin. Endothelial cells, which are more or less always involved in tissue damage, can express interleukins, chemokines, and the vasodilator nitric oxide.

These factors lead to the well-known cardinal signs of inflammation: swelling, redness, pain, heat, and ultimately loss of function (tumor, rubor, dolor, calor as the Roman physician Celsus so described it). In early inflammation, the capillary endothelium becomes porous and easy to transit. This floods the affected area with fluids. It will allow for neutrophils and ultimately lymphocytes (in a later wave of immune response) to use focal adhesion to move into the area to confront the threat. The inflammatory mediators signal to these other innate and adaptive immune cells, which can begin to arrive in minutes. This will be further reinforced as macrophages and dendritic cells absorb antigen (through phagocytosis for both but also through pinocytosis and membrane-mediated endocytosis for dendritic cells). Once antigen has been so processed, powerful cytokine signaling results, which orchestrates a more complex, secondary, adaptive, and ultimately specific immune response.

Cytokines in early inflammation include tumor necrosis factor-alpha (TNF-a) and interleukin beta1, which are secreted by macrophages and also, for TNF-a, mast cells. These signaling molecules will increase short-term inflammatory changes. MMP and proteolytic enzymes will be very active during inflammation, and this does cause destruction of localized ECM. This is part of the defense process. Resolution of inflammation occurs next. During resolution, interleukins such as IL-10 appear, which start to downregulate inflammation. This is followed by some rebuilding of ECM that was destroyed. Initially, a collagen scaffold is laid down by some fibroblasts, and this scaffold makes it easier for other fibroblasts to migrate to the area. The assembly of proteoglycans and attached glycosaminoglycans is followed by their decoration with the vesicles and sugars that are normally found there [2].

A notable extracellular matrix phenomenon occurs involving angiogenesis. During inflammation, the vascular endothelium opens up to allow white blood cells to walk into the ECM. This is called "Diapedesis," and it is governed by cytokines. This signal-driven diapedesis is known as chemotaxis. [3] Angiogenic factors are secreted during inflammation, driven by the presence of inflammatory mediators, the permeability of endothelium, which is enhanced by the exit of white blood cells, and the secretion of nitric oxide, a vasodilator. Vegetative endothelial growth factor (VEGF) is a blood vessel sprouting molecule secreted by macrophages, the endothelium itself, and other cells. VEGF causes a sprouting tip from the vascular endothelium near the site of inflammation to push out into the extracellular matrix. These sprouts can grow further to become branched blood vessels. This is a natural response to damaged tissue that is being rebuilt. The ECM itself can regulate this sprouting process. When matrix metalloproteinases cleave the ECM proteins, matricryptic sites are opened up. These are specific amino acid sequences in proteins that activate the sprouts from the endothelial cells and blood vessels to keep penetrating the area. For example, Arg-Gly-Asp (RGD) is a key matricryptic site that is found by the enzymatic cleavage of fibronectin. During resolution of inflammation, regression of unneeded blood vessel sprouts is steered by the ECM. If this fails to happen, excessive neovascularization can occur. This is found in some solid tumors, and in cases of post-inflammatory neovascularization of the cornea after wounds and infections.

In terms of resolution, the phenotypic switching of macrophages is key [4]. Macrophages can operate in M1 and M2 phenotypes. M1 phenotypes are associated with inflammation and MMP and generally protease activation. This is part of the normal anti-pathogen response, and it is destructive. It is spurred on by TNF-α, IL-1β, and IL-6, nitric oxide, and cyclooxygenase 2.

M2 phenotype macrophages are developed by IL-10, TFG-beta, and IL-4. This leads to less chemotaxis, less vasodilation, less white blood cell chemotaxis, and increased efferocytosis—the apoptosis and resorption of damaged cells.

Prostaglandins are one important kind of inflammatory mediator [5]. Originally discovered in seminal fluid, these are universal signaling molecules that have various species and functions. PGE2, for example, promotes inflammation and blood vessel permeability. PGE3 tends to be inflammation lowering. Prostaglandins are in fact formed by the metabolism of fatty acids. Certain fatty acids are acted on by enzyme systems. Arachidonic acid is key to the formation of pro-inflammatory PG2. Arachidonic acid is abundant in cell membranes. It is released by the enzyme phospholipase. It then is acted on by cyclooxygenase enzymes, to become inflammatory prostaglandins and thromboxanes, which increased platelet aggregation. By contrast, omega-3 fatty acids can create prostanoids with the opposite effect. Eicosapentaenoic acid leads to PG3 series that have little inflammation action and balance the pro-inflammatory PG1 series. They can also produce resolvins, which, as the name implies, resolve inflammation. Specifically, they can end the migration of white blood cells from the vascular system into the ECM. Docosapentaenoic acid, another omega-3 fatty acid, leads to the production of resolvins as well.

Therapy

Omega-3 and -6 Balance

A very common dietary fatty acid is linoleic acid. This is a 16-carbon omega-6 fatty acid. It is found in nuts, seeds, and meats. It is extremely prevalent in many diets due to the adoption of so-called seed oils. For instance, canola oil (made from rapeseed) is about 19% linoleic acid. Sunflower oil is about 29% linoleic acid. These omega-6 oils are converted in the body to arachidonic acid (AA), a 20-carbon omega-6 oil. AA is plentiful in the cell membrane, and it is used as a precursor for some of the key eicosanoids, which, as mentioned above, tend to be pro-inflammatory (Fig. 8.1). This is not intrinsically harmful as the entire suite of eicosanoids are part of the inflammatory-defense response.

The enzymes required to convert linoleic acid to AA are delta-6-desaturates, elongase, and delta-5-desaturase. These

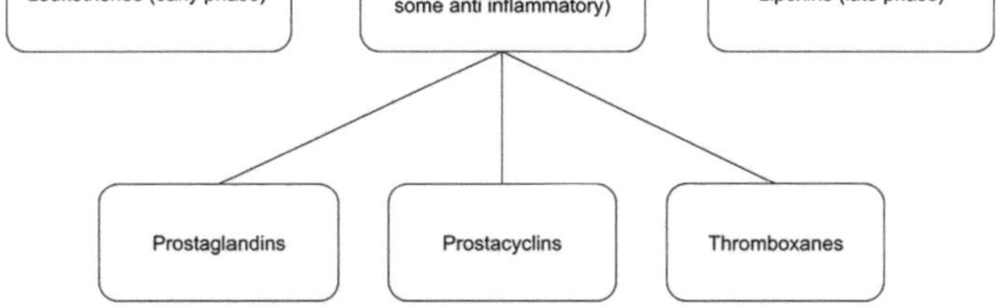

Fig. 8.1 Eicosanoids classification

same enzymes are also used in a different and equally important pathway (Fig. 8.2). Alpha-linolenic (ALA) acid is an omega-6 fatty acid found in plant foods such as walnuts, chia seeds, flax seeds, and avocado. Using the same enzyme sequence as linoleic acid, ALA can become eicosapentaenoic acid (EPA), a 20-carbon omega-3 fatty acid. EPA is a very important for a different series of eicosanoids that are inflammatory dampening and anticoagulant (Fig. 8.3). It can also be further elongated and desaturated to create docosahexaenoic acid (DHA), which also has anti-inflammatory pathways (and is important for brain and retinal development). EPA and DHA can also be obtained from fish, crustaceans, mollusks, and to lesser levels, some seaweeds [6–9].

In the early twentieth century, most people in the United States consumed more omega-3 s and far less omega-6 fatty acids [7]. Of course, poverty and malnutrition influenced the availability of omega-3 fatty acids, but, in general, the *ratio* of omega-6 to omega-3 in the diet was about 4:1 (Fig. 8.4). In contemporary America and developed countries in general, that ratio is 20:1.

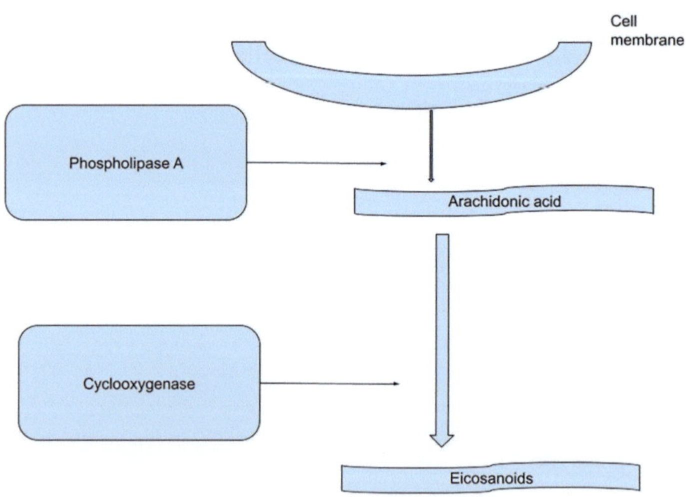

Fig. 8.2 Enzymes and eicosanoids

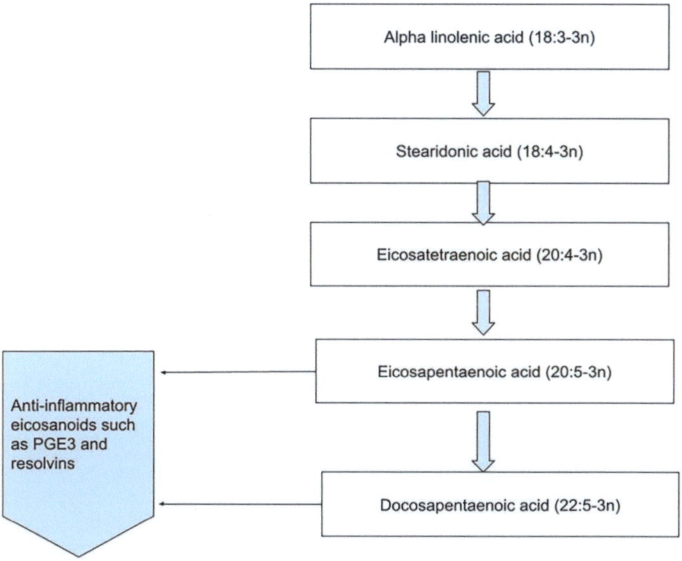

Fig. 8.3 Simplified omega-3 pathway

This is found through dietary surveys and backed up by linoleic acid levels found in tissue samples. Not only does this imbalance contribute to generalized inflammation, the severity of allergy, asthma, and autoimmune symptoms, and possibly neurological degeneration. These fatty acids use the same enzymes, and when there is an overwhelming dominance of linoleic acid, this further decreases the opportunities for the omega-3 pathway to create EPA and DHA from ALA.

With the goal of decreased ECM destruction due to overly exuberant inflammatory responses, the normalization of this ratio is important. This means a change in food choices to favor omega-3 sources, and a limitation of omega-6. This usually means a reduction in seed oils, which are rampant in processed food and restaurant food. There are additional downsides to these processed seed oils, which are discussed in the next chapter on deeper and chronic inflammation, but basically devolve upon oxidative stress and toxin exposure.

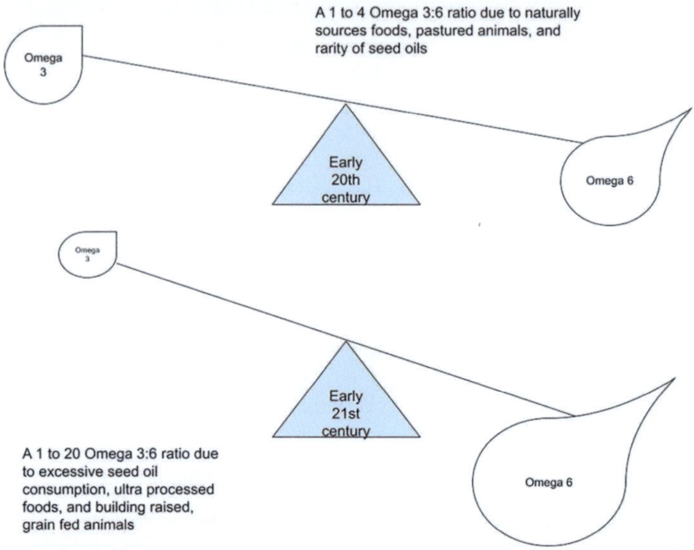

Fig. 8.4 Omega-3 and -6 balance

M2 Polarization

Macrophages are powerful drivers of immune and inflammatory activity. They have tissue-specific variants, for example, microglia in the brain, Kupfer cells in the liver, Langerhans cells in the skin, and pulmonary macrophages. Macrophages engulf and process antigen to T cells via major histocompatibility complex (MHC) I and II on their cell surface. Macrophages also have cell surface and cytoplasmic toll-like receptors and inflammasomes that can trigger innate immune responses. Macrophages can polarize, into what are referred to as M1 and M2 subtypes [4, 10, 11]. M1 types are pro-inflammatory and necessary for defense against pathogens and to sound the alarm in the presence of cancer cells. M2 polarities (and there are subtypes of these) are inflammation resolving. They promote healing and collagen deposition. In the extreme, M2 polarization can lead to immune system passivity in the face of cancer, or fibrosis due to excessive collagen deposition. In M1 dominance, overly exuberant inflammation can occur (Fig. 8.5).

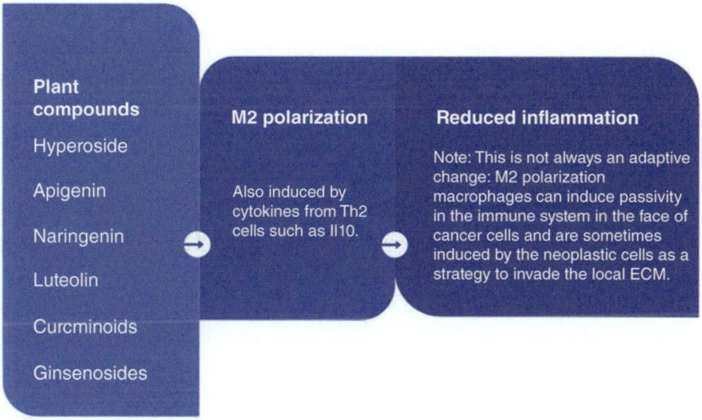

Fig. 8.5 Macrophage polarization

This polarization can reflect the polarization of T cells. Th1 lymphocytes are activators of CD8 T cells that have cytotoxic properties and are important for clearing the body of virus-infected cells and fighting neoplastic cells. Th2 polarization will activate antibody responses. Th1 cells secrete proinflammatory cytokines such as IL-12 and IFN-γ. Th2 cells secrete IL-4, IL-, and IL-10.

Plant extracts can encourage M2 polarization, which is sometimes desirable in the case of too much inflammation [10–12]. Examples include

Hyperoside, from *Rumex crispus* and *Drosera rotundifolia.*
Curcuminoids from *Curcuma longa.*
Apigenin from *Petroselinum crispum.*
Naringenin from grapefruit, oranges, and sour cherries.
Luteolin from T*araxacum officinale.*
Ginsenosides Rg3, Rb1, and Rg1 from *Panax ginseng.*

Plant Medicines That Decrease Inflammatory Prostanoids

Some plants used in herbal medicine have the ability to blunt the pathways that involve pro-inflammatory prostaglandins. One of these plants, *Salix alba* and *Salix nigra* (Willow bark) [13–15], is a source of salic acid, which was modified by the chemist Bayer in the nineteenth century to make acetylsalicylic acid, or aspirin. These plants appear to be easy on the gastrointestinal tract, a region that can become vulnerable to bleeding during the use of nonsteroidal anti-inflammatory drugs (NSAIDs) such as ibuprofen, naproxen, and aspirin. NSAIDs are very useful drugs, but from the naturopathic perspective, herbs such as actual willow bark are good for various acute inflammatory reactions including those of soft tissues and joints.

Ocimum sanctum (holy basil or tulsi) [16, 17] has a variety of anti-inflammatory sites in the body and decreases NFkB, a powerful driver of inflammation. It can improve cognition and mood, favorably impact metabolism and lipoproteins, and change inflammation in organs such as the lung and kidney.

Zingiber officinale or ginger has shoagals and gingerols, which can block cyclooxygenase and inhibit free radical formation [18]. Well known for anti-nausea functions, ginger also can be reduced in inflammation through the gastrointestinal tract and has some use in inflammatory bowel disease. It can also be found helpful in psoriasis, systemic lupus erythematosus, and rheumatoid arthritis.

Boswellia serrata or Frankincense is another good anti-inflammatory, especially for this level of dysfunction. It contains pentacyclic triterpenes—boswellic acids—which can reduce activity of 5-lipoxygenase and leukotriene B4 (LTB-4) [19–21]. It has a long history in traditional medicine and has been used to for skin and lung inflammations in many traditions in the Western Asia, the Mediterranean, and South Asia, where it is mostly grown. Using resins or balsams is a well-documented and ancient practice, and often, Frankincense was the resin of choice.

Harpagophytum procumbens or devil's claw is a plant native to Southeast Africa. It contains iridoid glycosides (harpagosides) and phenolic glycosides [22]. It has a reducing effect on inflammation of joints in particular and has been a popular natural medicine for arthritis for several decades. Overharvesting has threatened the plant, although cultivation has become more common. It can cause gastric upset for some patients.

Dietary and Therapeutic Oils

As noted above, the ratios of omega-3 to omega-6 have changed over the decades and become out of balance in many modern diets. The therapeutic use of omega-3 fatty acids has its place, both to create an anti-inflammatory effect by their ability to be precursors for anti-inflammatory eicosanoids, as well as rectifying an imbalance [9, 23–25]. Dietary balance is important too. There is nothing wrong with the presence of omega-6 in the diet but the sources should be mostly those which were not subject to ultraprocessing.

Examples of vegetable oils and their fatty acid profile [9]

Oil source	% Saturated	%Monounsaturated	% Omega-3	% Omega-6
Rapeseed	6.3	72.8	1.2[a]	19.6
Sunflower	18.2	28.3	0.2	62.2
Safflower	9.3	11.6	0.2	79.0
Peanut	10.7	71.1	0	18.2
Coconut	92.1	6.2	0	1.6
Olive	19.4	68.2	1.6	16.4
Sesame	16.9	43	0.2	40.9
Grape	10.4	14.8	0.2	74.7

[a] Hybridized "canola oil" will be higher in omega-3, closer to 8–10%

Dietary omega-3 sources [25]

Oil or food	EPA	DHA
Cod liver oil[a]	18.3	9.6
Halibut oil	9.6	30.6
Salmon oil	6.2	9.1
Skipjack tuna oil[b]	11	29.1
Shrimp	15.26	11.37
Lobster	17.04	7.69
Red crab	12.13	11.93
Squid	13.9	16.9
Surf clam	22.9	14.3
Icelandic scallop	26.9	25.9

[a]Being a liver oil will contain significant vitamin D and A, which has uses but also cautions for some populations, including pregnancy, where elevated vitamin A can be teratogenic

[b]Tuna oil must be filtered to remove toxins, especially mercury, which the fish accumulates

Supplemental omega-3 [25]

Omega-3 supplement	Dose	Remarks
Fish oil mixed EPA/DHA 2:1	1000 mg once a day to three times a day	Usually as fish oil concentrate where about $\frac{2}{3}$ of the oil is omega-3
DHA	400 mg once a day to twice a day	Useful for brain and retinal support, particularly in expecting mothers
Flax oil	1200 mg once a day to three times a day	Can also be consumed from bottled flax seed oil—Usually about 1 TBSP per day (kept refrigerated, and never used for frying that damages this oil very quickly)
Borage oil	1000 mg once per day	A non-marine source of essential fatty acids
Algae oil DHA/EPA 2:1	1000 mg once a day to twice a day	A non-marine source that is very high in omega-3
Evening primrose oil LA/ALA 1:1	1000 mg once a day to twice a day	Contains a fair amount of omega 6 but in a 1 to 1 ratio of linoleic acid to alpha-linolenic acid

Food sources of omega-3 [26]

Food	ALA amounts per 200 kcal (g)	Ratio of ALA to LA (omega-3 to omega-6)
Flax seeds	8.54	4:1
Chia seeds	7.34	3:1
Walnuts	2.78	1:4
Avocados	0.14	1:13

Anti-inflammatory plant extracts

Herbal medicine or extract	Mechanism	Dose	Remarks
Boswellia serrata [19–21]	Boswellic acids (pentacyclic triterpenes) inhibit proinflammatory cytokines, eicosanoids, elastases, and neutralize oxidative stress	400 mg three times a day—Standardized extract that contains 60% boswellic acids	Some preparations contain AKBA—Acetyl-11-keto-boswellic acid The preparations come from a resin obtained from the plant
Salix alba/Salix nigra [14]	Salicylic acid and its derivative salicin inhibit cyclooxygenase and reduce levels of pro-inflammatory prostaglandins and leukotrienes. May also reduce inflammatory cytokines	Tincture (hydro-ethanol extract) 3 ml once a day up to 4 times a day Capsules 500 mg once a day up to 4 times a day	May be standardized to 15% salicin. Effective inflammation changes but not as large an effect on blood coagulability as ASA (aspirin) Use with caution in those with history of peptic or duodenal ulcer
Ocimum sanctum (holy basil, tulsi) [16]	Phenolic compounds that prevent oxidative stress, particularly those caused by toxins such as aromatic carbon compound	Capsule of dried *Ocimum sanctum* 1 times a day to 3 times a day	Is also an adaptogen and has a long tradition in south Asian traditional medicine
Zingiber officinale (ginger) [18]	6-gingerol, which yields 6-shogaol from microbial metabolism and zingerone through internal metabolism have an anti-inflammatory effect. Acts as both a cyclooxygenase and lipoxygenase (5-LOX) inhibitor	500 mg once a day to three times a day	Has multiple health benefits, including improved digestion, decreases nausea, and chemopreventive properties

Herbal medicine or extract	Mechanism	Dose	Remarks
Harpagophytum procumbens [22]	Iridoid glycosides (harpagosides) and phenolic glycosides reduce inflammation via COX inhibition	Devil's claw root extract capsule 150 mg twice per day Tincture (water and ethanol extract) 3 ml twice per day	Will cause gastric upset for some patients—Not a good choice for those with very sensitive stomachs or current gastric pathology

References

1. Hannoodee S, Nasuruddin DN. Acute inflammatory response. PubMed. Treasure Island (FL): StatPearls Publishing; 2024. Available from: https://www.ncbi.nlm.nih.gov/books/NBK556083/
2. Arulselvan P, Fard MT, Tan WS, Gothai S, Fakurazi S, Norhaizan ME, et al. Role of antioxidants and natural products in inflammation. Oxidative Med Cell Longev. 2016;2016(5276130):1–15.
3. Arroyo AG, Iruela-Arispe ML. Extracellular matrix, inflammation, and the angiogenic response. Cardiovasc Res. 2010;86(2):226–35.
4. Liu YC, Zou XB, Chai YF, Yao YM. Macrophage polarization in inflammatory diseases. Int J Biol Sci. 2014;10(5):520–9.
5. Ricciotti E, FitzGerald GA. Prostaglandins and inflammation. Arterioscler Thromb Vasc Biol. 2011;31(5):986–1000.
6. Cholewski M, Tomczykowa M, Tomczyk M. A comprehensive review of chemistry, sources and bioavailability of Omega-3 fatty acids. Nutrients. 2018;10(11):1662.
7. DiNicolantonio JJ, O'Keefe J. The importance of maintaining a low Omega-6/Omega-3 ratio for reducing the risk of autoimmune diseases, asthma, and allergies. Mo Med. 2021;118(5):453.
8. Djuricic I, Calder PC. Beneficial outcomes of Omega-6 and Omega-3 polyunsaturated fatty acids on human health: an update for 2021. Nutrients. 2021;13(7):2421.
9. Orsavova J, Misurcova L, Ambrozova JV, Vicha R, Mlcek J. Fatty acids composition of vegetable oils and its contribution to dietary energy intake and dependence of cardiovascular mortality on dietary intake of fatty acids. Int J Mol Sci. 2015;16(6):12871–90.
10. Saqib U, Sarkar S, Suk K, Mohammad O, Baig MS, Savai R. Phytochemicals as modulators of M1-M2 macrophages in inflammation. Oncotarget. 2018;9(25):17937.
11. Im DS. Pro-resolving effect of Ginsenosides as an anti-inflammatory mechanism of Panax ginseng. Biomol Ther. 2020;10(3):444.

12. Liu J, Zhang Y, Sheng H, Liang CL, Liu H, Guerrero JM, et al. Hyperoside suppresses renal inflammation by regulating macrophage polarization in mice with type 2 diabetes mellitus. Front Immunol. 2021;12(12)
13. Willow Bark. PubMed. Bethesda (MD): National Library of Medicine (US); 2006. Available from: https://pubmed.ncbi.nlm.nih.gov/30000964/
14. Sharma S, Sahu D, Das HR, Sharma D. Amelioration of collagen-induced arthritis by Salix nigra bark extract via suppression of pro-inflammatory cytokines and oxidative stress. Food Chem Toxicol. 2011;49(12):3395–406.
15. Khayyal M, El-Ghazaly M, Abdallah D, Okpanyi S, Kelber O, Weiser D. Mechanisms involved in the anti-inflammatory effect of a standardized willow bark extract. Arzneimittelforschung. 2011;55(11):677–87.
16. Suresh A, Rao TC, Solanki S, Suresh MV, Menon B, Raghavendran K. The holy basil administration diminishes the NF-kB expression and protects alveolar epithelial cells from pneumonia infection through interferon gamma. Phytother Res. 2022;36(4):1822–35.
17. Cohen MM. Tulsi – Ocimum sanctum: a herb for all reasons. J Ayurveda Integr Med. 2014;5(4):251.
18. Ballester P, Cerdá B, Arcusa R, Marhuenda J, Yamedjeu K, Zafrilla P. Effect of ginger on inflammatory diseases. Molecules. 2022;27(21):7223.
19. Siddiqui MZ. Boswellia Serrata, a potential Antiinflammatory agent: an overview. Indian J Pharm Sci. 2011;73(3):255–61.
20. Majeed M, Majeed S, Narayanan NK, Nagabhushanam K. A pilot, randomized, double-blind, placebo-controlled trial to assess the safety and efficacy of a novel Boswellia serrata extract in the management of osteoarthritis of the knee. Phytother Res. 2019;33(5):1457–68.
21. Ammon H. Boswellic acids in chronic inflammatory diseases. Planta Med. 2006;72(12):1100–16.
22. Gxaba N, Manganyi MC. The fight against infection and pain: devil's claw (Harpagophytum procumbens) a rich source of anti-inflammatory activity: 2011–2022. Molecules. 2022;27(11):3637.
23. Holm Nielsen S, Sardar S, Siebuhr AS, Schlemmer A, Schmidt EB, Bay-Jensen AC, et al. Effect of n-3 PUFA on extracellular matrix protein turnover in patients with psoriatic arthritis: a randomized, double-blind, placebo-controlled trial. Rheumatol Int. 2021;41(6):1065–77.
24. Mariamenatu AH, Abdu EM. Overconsumption of Omega-6 polyunsaturated fatty acids (PUFAs) versus deficiency of Omega-3 PUFAs in modern-day diets: the disturbing factor for their "balanced antagonistic metabolic functions" in the human body. Kostner GM, editor. J Lipids. 2021;2021(1):1–15.
25. NCBI. F S, P A. Omega-3 Polyunsaturated Fatty Acids and Their Health Benefits. Annual review of food science and technology. 2018. Available from: https://pubmed.ncbi.nlm.nih.gov/29350557/
26. Myfooddata. Foods High in Alpha Linolenic Acid (ALA). myfooddata. Available from: https://www.myfooddata.com/articles/foods-high-in-ALA.php

Deeper Inflammation: Examples of Extracellular Matrix Involvement and Treatment

9

Inflammation will naturally occur in bursts whatever region of the body is facing infection or injury. This is the natural way to activate defenses and essentially remodel a tissue. Although acute inflammation can be so intense as to cause permanent disability or even death, most often it yields to resolution and healing. But inflammation can also become chronic. This can be a reaction to the decline of an organ and its necrosis. Or, the immune system can react to a certain tissue because of some autoimmune targeting of the tissue or a hypersensitivity reaction. Perhaps a pathogen has been contained, but not eliminated, and the infection and inflammation smolders away for months or years.

The mechanisms by which inflammation can become chronic and self-perpetuating have come into clearer focus. Moreover, the sorts of phenotypes and dietary imbalances that drive this type of inflammation are increasingly understood. One activator of this phenomenon are the advanced glycation end products–defective molecules that have a sugar bonded to them. Another example is the impact of environmental toxins and dietary toxins, and the consequences of depleting one's antioxidant enzyme pool.

The extracellular matrix is at the crossroads of inflammatory events [1]. Many of the components of innate immunity—complement, natural killer cells, macrophages—operate within the ECM. Successful innate immune responses against a pathogen are followed by adaptive immune responses. Although usually suc-

F. Smith, *The Extracellular Matrix in Health and Disease*,
https://doi.org/10.1007/978-3-031-94465-9_9

cessful, these will damage the ECM, in part by activating various proteases, including matrix metalloproteinases, and also through the oxidative stress created by white blood cell attacks on pathogens. The fragments of various ECM proteins in turn can be drivers of inflammation. This is true even in reasonably healthy ECM environments. But in aged, inflamed, and glycated matrix environments, inflammatory reactions are more intense, prolonged, and easily initiated.

The aspects of deeper inflammation mean that local innate immune defenses persist beyond an adaptive, beneficial time period. It also results in other aspects of the immune system, such as neutrophils, and eventually cytotoxic T cells, will migrate to the area and release-oxidizing compounds. Neutrophils will release destructive granules that are part of fighting bacteria, but these oxidative compounds will damage the matrix. Moreover, neutrophil elastase is a powerful enzyme that will shear elastin fibrils, causing elastin to fragment and unravel. So, while inflammation is an issue for cells in particular, it is a major determinant of extracellular matrix homeostasis. Just as nutrition and antioxidant defenses are a determinant of ECM structure and function, the regulation of inflammation is a major determinant.

Pattern Recognition Receptors

The scientists Charles Janeway and Ruslan Medzhitov, through innovative and painstaking research, discovered the toll system. Janeway had reinvigorated the research into a relatively ignored area of innate immunity in the 1980s. Janeway was looking for ways, some element, in innate immunity can activate adaptive immunity and elaborated the concept of pattern recognition receptors. Medzhitov, a grad student under Janeway, found the toll-like receptor in humans after seeing its function in other species [2].

Research on pattern recognition receptors (PRRs) has exploded, and the true clinical potential of these discoveries has only begun to be seen. PRRs are found in many innate immune cells, including macrophages, neutrophils, dendritic cells, and epithelial cells.

Toll-like receptors are a type of pattern recognition receptors (PRRs). These are molecular sensors that detect molecules that are formed during cell or extracellular matrix destruction. They can also detect the presence of destroyed pathogens, but they are not limited to sensing invading microorganisms. Very importantly, PRR will alert the rest of the immune system to damage to the organism's own cells and tissue matrix [3].

There are numerous molecular signals that can activate PRR. One very clinically significant type is the damage-associated molecular patterns (DAMPs) [4]. This includes fragments of DNA, histones, key chromosome proteins, mitochondrial proteins, and various extracellular matrix glycoproteins and fibrillar proteins. Although the organism's resources are used to mount responses to the presence of DAMPs, it must have served as a beneficial enough early warning system to have been evolutionarily conserved and is found in many species (Fig. 9.1).

Pathogen-associated molecular patterns (PAMPs) are derived from bacteria, protozoa, and viruses. This could be lipopolysac-

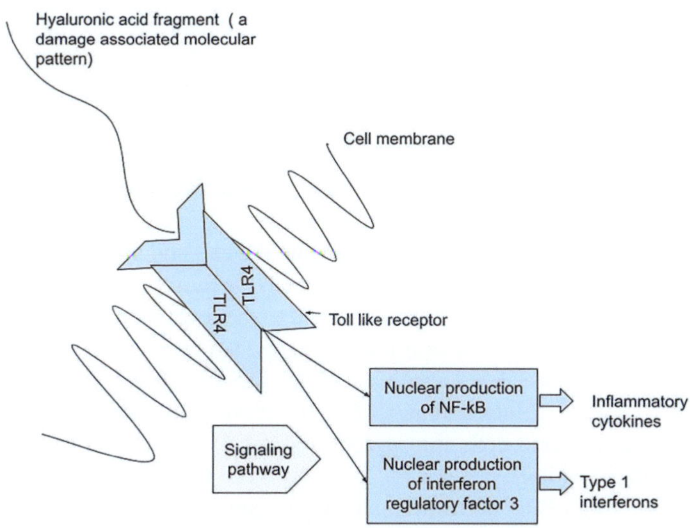

Fig. 9.1 Damage-associated molecular patterns and receptors

charides from gram-negative bacteria, lipoteichoic acid from gram-positive bacteria, and nonhuman nucleic acid motifs that are created by viruses. Although immune recognition of invaders has been a central concept in immunology since the beginning of the discipline, the idea that molecular motifs from self-damage and those from pathogens could bind to receptors comprising the same early warning system was completely novel [5].

There are numerous types of PRR. The first discovered, toll-like receptors (TLR) are comprised of TLR1 to TLR13 in humans. Some are found in the endosomal compartments inside the cell (these being TLR3, TLR7, TLR8, and TLR9) and the others [1, 2, 4–6, 10–13] are transmembrane. When a DAMP or PAMP binds to a toll-like receptor, it causes an adaptor to bind. TLR 1,2,4,5,6,7,8, and 9 use the adaptor MYD88 (myeloid differentiation primary response 88) and TLR 3 and 4 use TRIF (TIR-domain-containing adapter-inducing interferon-β, also known as TIR domain-containing adaptor molecule 1 or TCMA1).

Once these adaptors have activated, the TLR-adaptor complex will initiate a signaling pathway that leads to inflammatory responses. This includes the MAP kinase pathway (examples being ERK, p38, and JNK), the well-known NFkB pathway, and the IRF (interferon regulatory) factors pathway. These pathways lead to increased IL-6, TNF-alpha, and IL-12, which activate inflammatory responses, including the attraction of adaptive immune cells. There might also be IL-10 release, which is down-regulating inflammation.

NOD-like receptors are found inside the cell and effect similar responses. The NOD group includes the NLR family pyrin domain containing 3 (NLRP3). This is integral to the formation of inflammasomes, primarily within macrophages, which release caspase 1. When caspase 1 is created, it can lead to increased interleukin 1β (IL-1β) and interleukin 18 (IL-18) production and can push bacteria-infected cells into pyroptosis (a cell destruction caused by inflammation).

Although PRR activation is an important form of defense and tissue remodeling, it can get out of control. Ongoing DAMP production due to cell destruction in an inflammatory, infectious, or traumatic disease can continue to activate inflammation, which simply generates more DAMPs because cells or ECM are destroyed in the process. This can contribute to morbidity of some conditions, even those not considered primarily inflammation in nature, such as osteoarthritis. It can also drive clearly inflammatory conditions, such as steatohepatitis, into deeper levels of dysfunction. This can deteriorate to the point of becoming a positive feedback loop.

Advanced Glycation End Products (AGEs)

AGEs are formed by the reactions of sugars with proteins. This can happen during cooking (and a small percentage of AGE from food are absorbed), but also happens in the body. People with elevated blood glucose levels will produce more AGE. Twarda-Clapa et al. published a comprehensive overview of AGE in 2022 [6]. The multistep formation of AGE can follow Maillard or Polyol pathways leading to Amodori or Heynes products, respectively. These can lead to a series of reactive carbonyls, such as glyceraldehyde. These lead to a final form, the advanced glycation end products. These include

- Glucose-derived.
- Fructose-derived.
- Glyoxal-derived.
- Methylglyoxal-derived.
- Glyceraldehyde-derived.
- Glycolaldehyde-derived.
- 3-Deoxyglucosone-derived.

AGE can lead to aging and inflammation in three ways. They can stick to proteins and crosslink them. This leads to stiffer tissues, and in the case of the extracellular matrix, changes to stiffness changes mechanotransduction that impacts cell proliferation and migration. AGE can also generate oxidative stress, such as hydroxyl radicals and superoxide anions (Fig. 9.2).

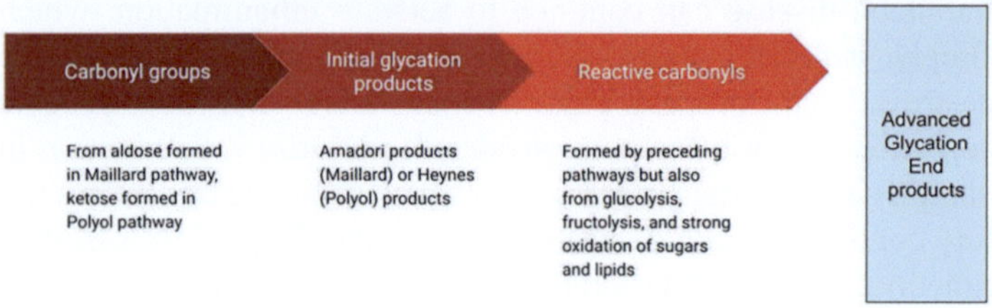

Fig. 9.2 Advanced glycation end products

Powerfully, AGE can bind to a particular receptor, known fittingly as the receptor for advanced glycation end products (RAGE). Although AGE can also bind to various scavenger receptors, RAGE is well known to provoke inflammation in its role as a pattern recognition receptor. This leads to an increase in inflammatory cytokines such as TNF-α, IL-1, and IL-6. There are soluble forms of RAGE, produced by the actions of ECM matrix metalloproteinases, that can blunt the binding of the typical AGE molecules to the transmembrane RAGE (receptor).

Inflammatory Phenotype

When a person has suffered years of oxidative stress beyond the ability of their normal antioxidant enzyme systems, augmented by various dietary phenols, flavonoids, and terpenes, their ECM changes. It becomes crosslinked and less functional. Ongoing damage can continue to provoke inflammation via the PRR system. Glycation of proteins, as noted above, will powerfully activate its own receptors, including RAGE, scavenger receptors, and some TLR. This will push macrophages into M1 modes, which are destructive and meant only for dealing with immediate infection or tissue remodeling issues. This in turn leads to more production of DAMPs, which of course bind to the PRR and create yet more inflammation. Due to the lack of dietary determinants of health, the overconsumption of pro-inflammatory dietary ingredients, an abundance of environmental toxins, possible self-administered toxins such as tobacco smoke or certain drugs of abuse, and dysregulated insulin receptors and blood sugar levels, will find themselves in a state of advanced aging. They will also be in a state of ongoing inflammation, which may wax and wane depending on the various stressors on the person, but never truly resolve. This may lead directly to certain disease states (such as neuropathy in a diabetic) or contribute to a myriad of other pathologies. In general terms, it is a state of permanent inflammation that promotes aging. The term "inflammaging" was coined by Italian scientists who have studied this phenomenon in depth [7]. Under such conditions, stem cells actually become unable to activate themselves, and these stem cells display senescent behaviors far beyond the chronological age. There is also excessive production of DAMPs and overactivation of PRR. This becomes a vicious cycle in such individuals. This senescence-associated secretory phenotype is a new target for therapy, not only because the causes can be lessened or eliminated, but because the senescent cells themselves block normal tissue repair [8].

Neuroinflammation

In multiple sclerosis, the immune attacks on the central nervous system lead to damaging amounts of inflammation. This leads to direct changes to the ECM. In health, there are distinct types of ECM in the brain [9]. There are of course basement membrane ECM structures in the endothelium of blood vessels, with certain modifications to make the brain rather immune privileged (the "blood–brain barrier"). The interstitial spaces between cells have chondroitin sulfate proteoglycans (CSPG) (Fig. 9.3). The bodies of neurons are surrounded by perineural nets and plenty of tenascin and hyaluronate bound to CSPGs. These neural nets are important for synaptic plasticity and repair. After immune attack, microglia become overactive and contribute to local inflammation. Excessive CSPG production leads to an imbalance of this type of molecule, an overabundance of what is normally a useful molecule in the brain ECM. This has a suppressive effect on oligodendrocyte cell (ODC) replacement. ODCs are cells that make the myelin that the CNS needs for normal conduction velocities.

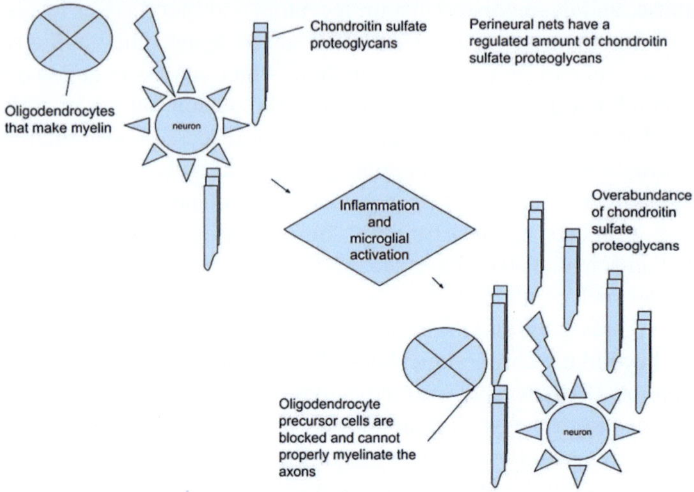

Fig. 9.3 Chondroitin sulfate proteoglycans and neuronal damage

With ODC suppression (and less myelin) due to improper ECM replacement, some areas of the CNS will remain myelin bare, which will manifest as MS symptoms. Moreover, various ECM molecules can act as DAMPs, which can lead to a smoldering inflammation.

The brain extracellular matrix is supportive of neuronal development, plasticity, and defense. One example of brain ECM are the perineural nets that surround some cells. Inflammation in the brain can be induced by oxidative stress, toxins, or infection. This can lead to the activation of protective microglial cells, which act as a resident scavenger and innate defense for the CNS. This leads to ECM remodeling, but too much or ongoing microglial activity can lead to ECM destruction and ultimately loss of function or degenerative changes in parts of the CNS. The brain does have its own pattern recognition receptors, including NOD receptors. Moreover, the gut's pattern recognition receptors can influence the CNS via cytokine release and nervous input via the vagus nerve. These gut changes can be dysbiosis or inflammatory disease as by Keough, Rude, and Gareau in their 2022 paper on this topic [10]. Thus, gut inflammation can activate microglia and lead to brain inflammation. The brain has its own Receptor for advanced glycation end products (RAGEs) so that glycated proteins and beta-amyloid (found in various neurodegenerative diseases including Alzheimer's disease) can bind to it. This binding causes neuroinflammation via the upregulation of NfKBeta and can do this both within the brain ECM and the vascular endothelium. The latter effect of RAGE activation will alter the vascular endothelium of the brain, including the nearby astrocyte foot projections and the tight junctions of the endothelium.

Cardiac Inflammation

The cardiac extracellular matrix is abundant in collagen, especially type 1. It provides structural integrity to a muscle that contracts constantly throughout life. This ECM wraps around myofibrillar bundles and has three layers, endomysium, perimysium, and epimysium. The endomysium is bound to the myofibrillar bundles via integrin, so shares a very tight connection with these cell bundles. Like the other layers, it provides structural support and alignment, keeping myofibrils properly oriented, and in the case of endomysium, to prevent distraction of the myofibrils and ventricular swelling. When inflammation in the heart is too intense, it disrupts this ECM, leading to less efficiency organization of myofibrils [11].

Lung Inflammation

The lung is replete with innate immune features, including mast cells. Various pathogens come into contact with the lung every day, and the tissue can also become sensitized to otherwise harmless agents such as pollen when allergy develops (typically at type 1 hypersensitivity). Irritants to the lung such as cigarette smoke or air pollution can also create damage. Damage to the epithelium and underlying parenchyma of the lung lead to fibroblast activation and efforts to remodel. Inflammatory signaling molecules and cytokines will be released, including platelet activity factor, bradykinin, and cytokines such as IL-1, TNF, and IL-6. These inflammatory responses can become too prolonged or exuberant. In the case of asthma, continued release of inflammatory compounds causes edema in the airways and increased hypersensitivity. This is always accompanied by changes to the ECM. Inflammation will lead to remodeling that can become ongoing, and instead of resolution, can lead to damage [12].

Renal Inflammation

Oxidative stress and resulting or concomitant inflammation will injure the kidney [13]. This injury creates reactive changes that can eventually lead to fibrosis. The kidney has its discrete structures within the basic filtration unit, the nephron. This includes mesangium, Bowman's capsule, capillary endothelium, and components of the tubules. These are all backed up by extracellular matrix, which needs to have the correct proportions and types of collagens and proteoglycans, and other molecules (such as versican, fibronectin, biglycan, and decorin). Inflammation in the kidney that is prolonged or intense will activate matrix metalloproteinases and lead to degradation of the ECM, and later, reactive collagen formation. There are many causes of renal inflammation including infection and autoimmune phenomena. The kidney does have toll-like receptors in the nephron, and therefore has the capacity for maladaptive innate immune responses.

Consequences of Inflammation

Although inflammation is an important protective and remodeling process, when it fails to become self-limiting, it will progress to pathology. The normal regulatory shut-offs for inflammation can be overwhelmed by upregulating signals from inflammation-damaged cells, extracellular matrix, and in infectious cases—pathogens. For the ECM, this means that excessive matrix metalloproteinase activation, and elastases, will degrade the structural integrity of the matrix. This causes immediate malfunctions in the nourishment and maintenance of cells. Moreover, the ECM, via its many connections to cells and their nuclei and mitochondria, is an important regulator of cell proliferation and migration. This loss of ECM integrity due to inflammatory destruction can impact the health of tissues [14, 15]. The progression of this process, the fate of tissues that are ravaged by inflammation and develop extensive ECM damage, is the focus of upcoming chapters. The self-propagating damage that veers toward a positive feedback versus a negative feedback control (or lack thereof) can be interrupted with the removal of the inflammation provoking factors. This is not always enough, and in addition to addressing longer term causative factors, changes to the inflammatory activity of the ECM and surrounding cells needs to be done. Although a deeply inflamed ECM is a serious matter, it is still part of an adaptive system that can, for a time, respond to modulators such as dietary factors, plant extracts, and hormetic (minute dose) inputs.

Dietary Considerations

Diet plays a major role in impacting inflammation. In the preceding chapter, the topic of diet and the propensity for inflammation were discussed. In terms of prevention of chronic inflammation and types of exuberant inflammation that becomes destructive, diet is equally important. This is due to many factors as diet can.

(a) Provide fatty acids and nutrients that support biochemical pathways that are inflammation resolving.
(b) Minimize the intake of pro-inflammatory and pro-oxidant foods.
(c) Be lower rather than higher on the NOVA classification.
(d) Influence the gut microbiome in ways that decrease inflammation throughout the body.
(e) Include foods that have compounds such as polyphenol that are anti-inflammatory.

There is no one approach to an anti-inflammatory diet that is known to be the best for everyone, and there is unlikely to be one. Individual genotypes and phenotypes will lead to differing nutritional requirements and levels of tolerance of dietary factors. A person's immune system as a product of their genetics, nutritional status, physiological functioning, and acquired hypersensitivities. Aside from individual differences, just the exact composition of a diet that is best is still becoming clearer as the science of human biochemistry and physiology advances. The very concept of "a diet" has inherent flaws as eating can be idiosyncratic based on preferences, lifestyle, culture, food preferences, socioeconomic factors, and simple availability of food (seafood might be easier to come by near the ocean, tropical fruits might not be readily available in all temperate zones).

(a) Provide Fatty Acids and Nutrients That Support Biochemical Pathways That Are Inflammation Resolving

As discussed in the preceding chapter, the intake of adequate omega-3 fatty acids and a correct ratio of omega-3 to omega-6 fatty acids in the diet are important [16]. That ratio should be closer to 1:4 and not the 1:20 that is seen in many developed countries. A proper amount of omega-3 fats leads to the production of eicosanoids that help modulate and contain inflammation.

The support of the intrinsic antioxidant systems is important for decreasing the damage that can result from innate immune responses [17, 18]. This includes amino acids glycine and cysteine, and zinc, the B vitamins, including methylfolate, vitamin E, and vitamin C. The building up for glutathione levels not only mops up free radicals and might help prevent vicious circles of inflammation; it plays a role in Th balance in immunity. Naive T cells will differentiate into subsets. Th1 cells will secrete cytokines that direct cellular immunity, including cytotoxic T cells. Th2 cells will drive B cell activity and increase antibody responses. Treg cells have a moderating effect on inflammation and decrease hypersensitivity. Th17 cells are pro-inflammatory and tend to be involved in diseases such as inflammatory bowel disease. When glutathione levels in a T cell are low, it will tend toward Th2 differentiation, which will encourage inflammatory innate immune responses [19]. This is dynamic balance; all phases of a T cell have their purpose. But in a toxin-rich environment and under conditions of continuous oxidative stress, glutathione can become depleted.

(b) What Constitutes "Pro-Inflammatory" Ranges from Easy to Establish Dietary Factors to More Contestable, or Simply, Contextual Ones

Foods that are burnt contain heterocyclic amines and polycyclic aromatic hydrocarbons. [20] These molecules are found by the high heat reaction of amino acids, sugars, and creatine. The prime example is to grill a food at time temperature, where polycyclic aromatic hydrocarbons form when fats drip down onto the heat source and then evaporate or contact the food. Very high heat can create these molecules and is the factor in creating heterocyclic amines. These are believed to increase cancer risk, based on animal studies but not conclusively proven in humans. Such compounds are absorbed from the gut and then find their way to the liver. When they are processed by cytochrome P450 (phase 1 of detoxification), they become very reactive molecules. This enhanced oxidative product has to be neutralized by a phase 2 conjugate. In the process, antioxidants such as glutathione (which might also be used as the conjugate), vitamin C, and polyphenols from the diet need to be present to prevent damage to surrounding cell components. There is no established limit as to how many times per day or week a person can use high heat cooking before increasing oxidative stress and inflammation. Also of note is that ascorbic acid neutralizes the aromatic hydrocarbons as does increased amounts of fruits and vegetables in the diet. A meal with a protein seared on a hot grill, along with coleslaw and fruit, would have less oxidative impact. Conversely, a diet that had a lot of high heat-cooked proteins and lacked fruits, vegetables, vitamin C, and magnesium (which is not uncommon) would have oxidative stresses created by the actions of these heat-derived compounds and their metabolites.

A topic under investigation is that of seed-derived oils. This was mentioned in the preceding chapter from an omega-6 to omega-3 balance standpoint. The term seed oil refers to fatty acid extracts from soy, corn, sunflower, safflower, cottonseed, rapeseed, etc. Some of these oils, a small percentage of those consumed, are made by simply pressing the oil from these legumes and seeds. This of course leaves some fatty acids behind. Far more commonly, these oils are created at a literal industrial level. The seed is crushed and de-husked. It is pressed and then to remove additional fats, a solvent such as hexane is used, which maximizes oil extraction but must be removed because it is poisonous to humans. The hexane is evaporated, a process that involves heat [21–23]. The oil is then bleached and deodorized. There is also a step called winterization, which removes waxes from the oil so that when refrigerated it does not crystalize. That is a hallmark of oils such as true extra virgin olive oil. The concern with this process is twofold. One is the production of free radicals due to heat and chemical exposure, an example being peroxides. The processing can also remove, or expend, the natural antioxidants in the oil, particularly the tocopherols. According to the Pew Research Center, Americans on average consume 36 pounds of cooking oils per year—more than three times as much as in the early 1970s [24]. About 23% of calories in the diet come from these oils. This is unprecedented in American, and in fact, human diets. Although vegetable oils can have essential nutrients in them and can have positive health effects, eaten ad libitum, they seem capable of accelerating oxidative stress and inflammation.

Moderate or small amounts of vegetable oils within a diet that contains plentiful antioxidants and many stable fats such as olive oil and butter will have a modest contribution to the body's oxidative stress. This is even less significant if those oils are not used for cooking (which would subject them to heat, light, and oxygen and generate many free radicals). But when these oils become the central pillar of energy, flavor, and cooking in the diet, they simply contribute too many oxidized or oxidizable compounds with too little accompanying antioxidants (such as natural tocopherols found ubiquitously in oils or more food-specific antioxidants such as hydroxytyrosol: in olive oil). This unfortunate choice is made possible by the availability and sometimes near unavoidability (depending on where one eats) of ultraprocessed foods. The public health discussion on this topic is marred by the framing of the issue as either wholesale acceptance of vegetable oils as unconditionally healthy, or their condemnation of always harmful, neither of which seems to be the case.

(c) NOVA Classification

Examining a person's diet in terms of grams of carbohydrate, fat, and protein intake and the relative proportions of each has utility. Humans need certain amounts of macronutrients to be healthy. But this strictly quantitative approach has limits when considering the nature of the sources of those macronutrients. The NOVA classification was developed in Brazil and has been widely adopted. Both clinical trials and larger population observational research have confirmed its usefulness. The NOVA classification puts foods on a scale of I–IV. Group I are natural foods in an unadulterated state for minimally processed. They should not have added oils or chemicals [25]. Pasta made from milling wheat and then conditioning it with water can still be group I, and legume, fruits, and vegetables certainly are group II and relatively minimally processed, but are mostly condiments or culinary ingredients such as oils, vinegars, and honey, etc. Group III are processed foods, which have a particular meaning in NOVA, and include cheeses, breads, and canned food. Group IV are the ultra-processed foods, which are usually a product of an industrial food setting and have an alternated food matrix, many different kinds of additives from corn syrup to synthetic flavors, and are often complex amalgamations of many food extracts. These are not recipes in the traditional sense, but laboratory and factory creations that might require special production methods and sometimes rather sophisticated food chemistry.

Overconsumption of ultraprocessed foods is associated with many poor health outcomes, including cardiovascular disease, increased cancer risk, and neurological aging [26–28]. In the United

States, ultraprocessed foods comprised 57.9% of energy intake and contributed 89.7% of the energy intake from added sugars. By virtue of their additives and their displacement of lower NOVA scale foods in the diet, the IV/ultraprocessed foods can be said to be pro-inflammatory. Some are clearly so, such as potato chips made in cottonseed oil, sweetened breakfast cereals with artificial colors, or "granola" bars with high amounts of high-fructose corn syrup.

There are other classifications that have similar themes, distinguishing between processed and not processed. Pereira de Araújo et al. [29] made an excellent comparison of these systems in a 2022 review. The utility of these classification systems alongside dietary recommendations, such as myplate.gov in the United States, has been studied as well. It appears to be helpful to use NOVA as a tool. A person eating according to the latest guidelines, which emphasizes plant foods even more, and sets limits on added sugar, is almost certainly eating low on the NOVA classification. The question then arises, why should patients not just follow the dietary guidelines? And for some, this is all they need. But for practitioners and researchers, the NOVA scale and similar constructs speak to the actual eating, shopping, and cooking realities for our society. The shopper carts in many grocery stores or the bags left on many porches are replete with ultraprocessed items. Some of these even have some virtues; they might deliver a nutrient a person needs by virtue of being fortified with it (such as a chocolate milk beverage that has a day's worth of vitamin D for a child). But when these foods *become* the diet, new problems arise. A palate and really a brain that is accustomed to instant satisfaction from highly engineered and heavily processed foods may not make room for all of the excellent choices in the guidelines. People are surrounded by ultraprocessed foods from birth to old age, and 1 in 3 Americans purchases "fast food" every day.

Moreover, there are diminishing returns from an overly reductionist approach to food and eating. Most certainly, an analytic and quantitative approach to nutrition is a requirement for it to be a scientific enterprise. In many clinical situations, a quantitative approach to caloric intake, protein, fats, and various micronutrients is needed for a plan of care. Nutrition researchers and practitioners think a lot about how this biochemical knowledge translates into foods and meals. But eating can become overly complex. People with low or even moderate education in biochemistry, physiology, food science, and medicine can easily become confused by an overly reductionist approach. Should they eat 10% of their calories from protein for 40%? How much vitamin D do they really need? If all foods are just collections of digestive molecules, does it really matter where I get my nutrients from?

This kind of thinking, which is fostered in the public by daily press release about this or that study, massive amounts of advertising for food "products," a lifelong exposure to ultraprocessed and fast food and highly preprepared restaurant food, proclamations by experts of different kinds, and various social media opinions and trends, leads to inaction. Inaction leads to gravitation toward what is easy, familiar, sometimes cheap, and rather addictive, that being ultraprocessed food.

When people choose simple, unadulterated whole foods, they are bypassing a range of issues and decisions. Many traditional societies have done just fine eating a variety of local, seasonal, and unadulterated foods. An example in the more affluent world of advanced economies can be found in France. There is a country that produces much locally or small farm food, and people eat a variety of low NOVA options (Fig. 9.4). Portion size and lack of fast foods have been working for the French for some time. This

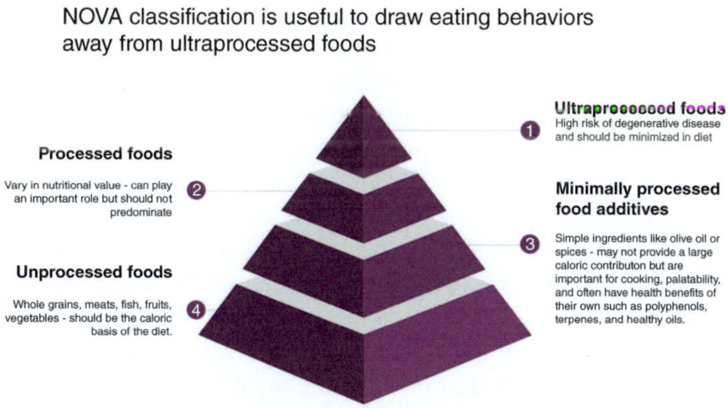

Fig. 9.4 NOVA classification

is shifting somewhat due to the intrusion of ultraprocessed foods found at the local corner store or the fast food outlet.

A diet that is strong on fundamentals can include some ultraprocessed food. But this must be handled carefully. The percentage of the food supply that is ultraprocessed foods in the United States is 73% [30]. This is entirely unacceptable and is contributing to massive health issues such as obesity, diabetes, stroke, heart disease, and undoubtedly neuroinflammation and mood disorders. Just because an ultraprocessed food may have some nutrient density, or that some low-processed foods are lower density, does not abolish the importance of simple, varied, eating in a way similar to natural human diets and in modern times, cultures such as France. Other food guidelines, and other major issues, such as food access, will continue to be important.

(d) Food and the Gut Microbiome

Diet is a major determinant of the composition, diversity, and behavior of the gut microbiome. Since food is medium for growth of these microorganisms, it is a necessary and rate-limiting factor. But the relationship here is complex. Some food ingredients will have compounds that suppress certain bacteria. The food compounds are not necessarily wholly consumed by microorganisms, and in the case of bacteria, may be simply transformed by the microbiota. Thus, dietary ingredients become substrates for chemical reactions whose products can impact host physiology. An example would be a compound called Equol, which is formed when gut bacteria metabolize a bioflavonoid from soy called daidzein. Equol is a rather strong phytoestrogen, and it is also anti-inflammatory. Another example would be sucralose, a net-zero sweetener. Although sucralose is not a source of energy for humans, bacteria can metabolize it. In a mouse model study, sucralose ingestion at an amount comparable to a human daily intake caused shifts in the microbiota of the mice leading to a change in the animal's gene expression toward a more inflammatory state.

Saturated Fats

This source of energy has been much maligned, and while overconsumption of saturated fats can lead to changes in physiology and increased health risks, there is a crucial issue at the heart of this issue. A great deal of what saturated fats mean for a person's health depends upon the kinds of foods in general that they consume. Saturated fat intake can increase the gut levels of lipopolysaccharide (LPS), a component of the cell wells of gram-negative bacteria [31–33]. LPS has a core of sugars with polysaccharides on one end of the molecule and fatty acids on the other. Many components of bacteria of all kinds, including gram-positive bacteria, can activate pattern recognition receptors including toll-like receptors. But LPS is particularly potent at activating inflammatory responses. This can provoke local inflammation in the gut, which can increase gut permeability and lead to more absorption of the breakdown products of food (putrefactive products) and various bacterial, archaeal, viral, fungal, and protozoal antigens. The gut has a fairly effective barrier in prevent overwash from antigens and direct invasion by the microbiota. Cells in the colonic epithelium are bound together (from apical/ superficial to basal/deep) by tight junctions, E-cadehrin, and desmosomes. LPS will damage the tight junction molecules. These molecules at the apical aspect of gut epithelial connections are comprised of claudins and junctional adhesion molecules, which are (membrane) protein binding, and zonula occludens (ZOs), which connects the junction created by the two other proteins to the actin skeleton. Although tight junctions are not directly connected to the ECM, the actin skeleton of a cell in general is via many integrin linkages.

Saturated fat can come from a variety of sources. The term standard American diet is used to denote a high consumption of nonnatural foods. Since dietary customs, regionally, ethnically, and economically cause quite a bit of divergence in what that "standard" is, it is more productive to focus on the common denominator. This is a diet that focuses on the highest NOVA classification, that of *ultraprocessed* food. In such a diet, there is a lack of dietary fiber and fermented foods. Dietary fibers, such as cellulose or pectins, are converted to beneficial short-chain fatty acids (SCFAs) [34]: butyrate, acetate, propionate, etc. These SCFAs are a primary energy source of the colonic epithelium and, when present, help with better junctional integrity. Moreover, SCFAs, butyrate in particular, are anti-inflammatory to the gut. Dietary fiber alone is good, but really needs the correct microbial species to maximize its benefits.

Fermented Foods

Fermented foods are a constant in almost all traditional diets. Cuamatzin-Garcia et al., [35] in a comprehensive review of the effects of fermented foods on gut health, note the importance of prebiotic substances (oligosaccharides from dietary fiber sources but also beta-glycans from foods such as oats). Examples of traditional fermented foods in the article, which is just a sample of many culinary traditions, are

- Yogurt.
- Cheeses.
- Crème fraiche.
- Fermented sausages.
- Sourdough bread.
- Soy sauce (brewed the traditional way—not soy protein isolate, caramel-colored "Soy Sauce").
- Fish sauce.
- Fermented vegetables, including "miso" (fermented soybeans), "kimchi" (fermented spicy cabbage), "sauerkraut" (fermented cabbage).
- "Surströmming" (fermented herring)
- "Kefir" (fermented milk)
- "Kombucha" (fermented tea)
- Beer, wine, or "kvass" (depends on products and ferment).
- Chicha—a corn ferment.
- Iru (fermented locust bean).
- Ogi (fermented cassava).
- Mabisi/Amasi (fermented milk).

These foods have their own prebiotics and many beneficial bacteria [36–39]. Some traditional diets obtain double-digit percentages of calories from such foods. The regular consumption of these foods, as is the norm in traditional and very often the lower on the NOVA classification diets, will have an anti-inflammatory effect on the gut. Conversely, those eating ultraprocessed diets will generally lack this protective aspect. Additionally, those ultraprocessed foods tend to have pro-inflammatory properties, such as a highly exaggerated omega-6 to −3 ratio, many chemical-damaged fats (reducing the potential benefits of polyunsaturated fatty acids), extreme amounts of high-fructose corn syrup, food dyes that have been banned in many countries, excessive amounts of added sugars in a food matrix (or lack thereof) guaranteed to make that good very high in the glycemic index, and an assortment of processing chemicals, some of which are fairly benign (potassium sorbate) and others that do not belong in the human diet (propylparaben). The lack of antioxidants, including plant compounds such as carotenoids and polyphenols in the ultraprocessed diet, has general and gut-specific effects. Inflammation is less easily quenched in the absence of these free radical-scavenging compounds.

(e) Food Compounds That Are Generally Protective of the Extracellular Matrix

As important as the gut is for human health, thinking more broadly about the impact of diet in the actual tissues, and specifically in the ECM, is important. Certain nutrients that have an established estimated average required are a part of the ECM protection. But it is also necessary, or at least highly desirable, to consume plant compounds that protect the ECM in order to avoid that sustained inflammation that will lead to its eventual degeneration.

Additional Biochemical Support

Polyphenols are compounds found abundantly in many plants, including fruits and vegetables that humans consume (Fig. 9.5) [40, 41]. They contain phenolic rings and hydroxyl groups. There are flavonoid and nonflavonoid types of polyphenols. The nonflavonoids category includes

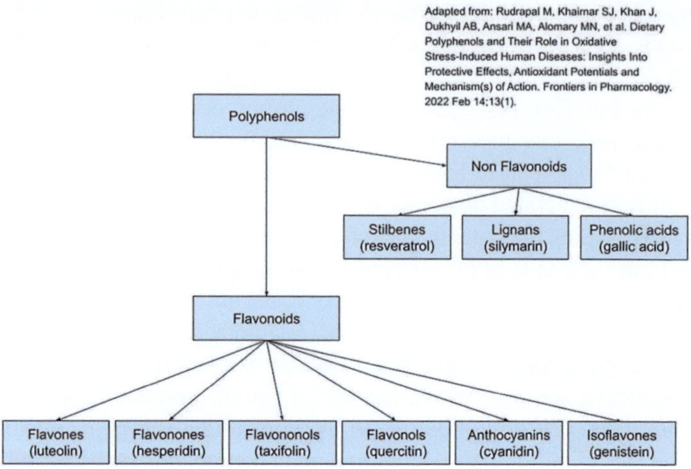

Fig. 9.5 Polyphenols [41]

- Phenolic acids (gallic acid).
- Stilbenes (resveratrol).
- Lignans (silymarin).

The flavonoid category includes

- Flavones (luteolin).
- Flavonones (naragenin).
- Flavonols (quercetin).
- Flavononols (taxifoln).
- Anthocyanins (cyanidin).
- Isoflavones (genistein).

These compounds have an amazing array of effects, some being very specific to certain receptors and tissues. For example, genistein is well known as a selective estrogen receptor modulator. Resveratrol, as we shall see in a later chapter, has chemopreventive and helpful effects in the tumor microenvironment.

In terms of the pervasive inflammation that can destroy the extracellular matrix and create an environment for cells that is inimical to healthy function, polyphenols exhibit a wide array of effects.

Polyphenols are directly antioxidant as they scavenge free radicals effectively. They also can chelate some metal ions that can act as catalysts for free radical generation—such as iron and copper.

Blunt the Activation of Inflammation due to Pattern Recognition Receptor Binding

Some polyphenols, such as those from *Curcuma longa* (turmeric), can downregulate the expression of certain toll-like receptors. Polyphenols can also downregulate cytokine expression, particularly the proinflammatory cytokines TNF-alpha and IL-6.

Even if PRR such as toll-like receptors are bound, polyphenols can decrease the downstream effects. They can interfere with activation of MAPK (mitogen-activated protein kinase), and suppress expression of NFkB, a powerful inducer of inflammation.

Polyphenols also decrease the production of inflammatory prostaglandins by suppressing the enzymes phospholipase A2 (PLA2), cyclooxygenase (COX), and lipoxygenase (LOX) .

They may increase the availability of the intrinsic antioxidant enzymes superoxide dismutase and catalase, and increase intracellular glutathione.

In the ECM, polyphenols seem to prevent excessive crosslinking of collagens. This is by controlling overactivation of lysyl-oxidase enzymes, which have their normal function, but can create too rigid a matrix. Conversely, the dampening of inflammation and oxidative stress will decrease macrophage release of matrix metalloproteinase, which can lead to too much destruction of the ECM.

Specific Probiotics That Target Inflammation

Generally, a gut flora that are diverse and supported by a diet that has natural fermented foods, plentiful dietary fiber, and plant foods will function normally. This is not always the case, however, and stress, toxins, and medications, in particular antibiotics, can alter the microflora. Adak and Khan outlined the microbial composition of the human gut in a 2019 paper in *Cellular and Molecular Life Sciences* [42]. The gut has local preponderance of bacteria in stomach, small bowel, large bowel, etc., but in general is inhabited by Firmicutes, Bacteroidetes, Actinobacteria, Fusobacteria, Proteobacteria, Verrucomicrobia, and Cyanobacteria.

Gut flora, as noted, enhance barrier integrity, regulate immune activity, and support normal metabolic function.

Gut bacteria can take dietary choline (meat being a good source) and convert them into trimethylamine, which is absorbed into the portal circulation, and in the liver, flavin monooxygenase converts it to trimethylamine N-oxide (TMAO), which has very proinflammatory actions, particularly on the vascular wall. TMAO can also provoke hypertension and disturb the electrical function of the heart. As noted above, lipopolysaccharides (LPS) form but metabolize fatty acids can be broadly proinflammatory in the body and locally in the gut. Phenylacetylglutamine, a gut product of the amino acid phenylalanine, is associated with serious cardiac and cerebrovascular events.

Patients with atherosclerosis had a significant increase in the abundance of *Escherichia coli, Klebsiella* spp., and *Enterobacter aerogenes*, and a decrease in the abundance of two butyric acid-producing bacteria, *Roseburia gutis* and *Faecalibacterium* cf. *prausnitzii* [43].

These atherosclerotic events are inflammatory in nature, driven by cytokine activation, and rooted in inflammasome and other pattern recognition receptor responses to these toxins. There are numerous beneficial microbial species and strains, and as stated above, diversity and stability of physiologically compatible and often symbiotic microbiota is the goal. Some species have been found to be specifically anti-inflammatory to the cardiovascular system. These include

- *Lactobacillus fermentum.*
- *Bifidobacterium animalis.*
- *Bifidobacterium breve.*

These probiotics have been found to lower inflammatory cytokines in humans such as TNF-alpha and increase endothelial healthy function, which will include the ECM projection of the endothelial glycocalyx.

Also useful are the commonly supplemented *Lactobacillus acidophilus, Lactobacillus reuteri, Lactobacillus fermentum, and Bifidobacterium bifidum.*

Some probiotics have been found to encourage M1 to M2 polarization in macrophages. As noted above, M1 macrophages are more active in promoting inflammation, and in the ECM this includes the commonly used *Lactobacillus acidophilus* as well as *Bacillus subtilis* (a gram-positive, spore-forming bacteria) [44, 45].

Endocannabinoid System

This bodywise system was discovered to be responsive to extracts of *Cannabis sativa* but has its own intrinsic activators, the endogenous cannabinoids (i.e., anandamide). There are two basic types of endocannabinoid receptors: CB1 and CB2 [46, 47]. They are not confined to one body system but CB1 is concentrated in the central nervous system and CB2 in the periphery including the immune system. Endocannabinoid binding can stimulate adenosine monophosphate protein kinase (AMPK). This reduces the stimulation of the mammalian target of rapamycin complex 1 (mTORC1) on inflammasome assembly. This will in turn reduce inflammasome creation (via less NLRP3 activity). The importance of the endocannabinoid receptor will be further explored in the chapter on fibrosis, but it can have an anti-inflammatory effect and block the activation of inflammasomes resulting from DAMP or PAMP recognition.

CBD isolate is just cannabidiol, which has relaxing, anxiolytic, and anti-inflammatory properties. It lacks the compound THC, which has stronger psychoactive effects. Broad-spectrum CBD has terpenes, a class of compounds often associated with essential oils, but in fact a very large family of compounds. Terpenes can exert anti-inflammatory effects. Broad-spectrum CBD also does not have tetrahydrocannabinol (THC).

Erigeron Breviscapus

This plant has a long use in traditional Chinese medicine [48]. It is related to Philadelphia Fleabane (*Erigeron philadelphicus*). It contains flavonoids such as scutellarin, breviscapine, baicalin, quercetin, and luteolin; caffeoylquinic acid such as caffeic acid, 3-O-caffeoylquinic acid, dicaffeoylquinic acid, and tricaffeoylquinic acid; pyranone such as pyranside; and steroid compounds such as xylocone and epigenol. It has neuroprotective and anti-neuroinflammation effects. It reduces NFkB and can reduce Tau protein and beta-amyloid in the brain. It reduces inflammation in the brain vascular endothelium. Cultivated *Erigeron breviscapus* should be used as wild varieties are at risk.

Rosmarinus Officinale

Rosemary is a popular culinary herb but is rich in phenolic compounds and has both antiseptic, antispasmodic, and anti-inflammatory effects [49]. In addition to the antioxidant effects from diterpenes, there is also direct anti-inflammatory effects from diterpenes compounds, including carnosic acid and carnosol. These compounds can inhibit NF-κB, MAPK, Nrf2, SIRT1, STAT3, and NLRP3 inflammasomes.

Cordyceps Militaris

This fungus is used as a dietary supplement for immune support. Edible and medicinal fungi can work to activate immune responses but also to moderate them [50]. *Cordyceps militaris* has reduced NFkB release from cells in the presence of lipopolysaccharide. This is thought to be due to the glucan –β-D-Glcp (1 → 3)-linked.

Hormetic Effects

Small doses of provocative compounds that might cause irritation in larger amounts, but in microgram or low milligram amounts leads to reduction in inflammation. This is a hormetic effect, where some doses, between 0 and the beginning of possible adverse effects (often in the very middle of that range) display an effect that is opposite the higher (and usually better known) dose effects.

Traumeel, and similar products, contain very low doses of herbs and minerals. Some of these are known to be soothing and nutrition, while others are irritating and pro-inflammatory or even toxic in higher doses. Traumeel has been found to reduce inflammation, including lipoxygenase formation, by inducing the production of specialized pro-resolving mediators [51].

This medicine contains.

Aconitum napellus 2× 1.32 μl 5.22×
Arnica montana, radix 2× 2.20 μl 5.00×
Bellis perennis 2× 1.10 μl 5.30×
Belladonna 2× 2.20 μl 5.00×
Calendula officinalis 2× 2.20 μl 5.00×
Chamomilla 3× 2.20 μl 6.00×
Echinacea 2× 0.55 μl 5.60×
Echinacea purpurea 2× 0.55 μl 5.60×
Hamamelis virginiana 1× 0.22 μl 5.00×
Hepar sulphuris calcareum 6× 2.20 μl 9.00×
Hypericum perforatum 2× 0.66 μl 5.52×
Mercurius solubilis 6× 1.10 μl 9.30×
Millefolium 3× 2.20 μl 6.00×
Symphytum officinale 6× 2.20 μl 9.00×

It is likely that at these doses some hormetic effect is observed. This type of medicine is often used topically, but is also taken internally via tablets or drinkable solutions from an ampule.

Anti-inflammatory polyphenols: flavonoid and nonflavonoid types [41, 54, 55]

Polyphenol	Mechanism	Dose	Remarks
Apigenin [41]	Has protection against neuroinflammation: Reduce proinflammatory cytokines, attenuation of microglia activation, increase memory and repair enzymes p-CREB, and BDNF, downregulation of NLRP3 inflammasome, iNOS and COX-2 expression, reduction of toll-like receptor-4 expression and inhibition of nuclear factor-kappa B (NF-kB) activation. https://doi.org/10.1007/s10787-024-01538-4	Actual dose not known but supplements maybe have 50 mg or more: Food sources are fresh parsley, vine spinach, celery seed, green celery heart, Chinese celery, and dried oregano, thyme, and chamomile	Not limited to CNS—Has antidiabetic and antimicrobial effects
Luteolin [40, 41]	Decreases levels of IL-17 and suppress NFkB.	100 mg per day; often combined with other similar compounds *Taraxacum officinale* is a good source	Luteolin has known chemopreventive actions
Caffeic acid [40, 41]	Strong antioxidant. Can block IL-6 and TNF-a; in the brain can block beta-amyloid and tau protein accumulation (animal models).	Not clearly defined. In animal studies, very high dose are used such as 50 mg/kg. Coffee drinkers obtain about 200 mg per day Found in coffee, red wine, and black chokeberries as well as apples, plums, lingonberries, black chokeberries, and many herbs of the mint family, e.g., sage, thyme, oregano, marjoram, oregano, or spearmint	Beyond anti-inflammatory effects—Caffeic acid has many chemopreventive effects across different tissues as well as antidiabetic effects

Baicalin [41]	Via NRF2 activation, increases in glutathione peroxidase (GSH-PX), superoxide dismutase (SOD) and catalase (CAT). In a kidney model: Reductions in mRNA levels of pro-inflammatory cytokines (IL-1β, IL-6, MCP-1, and TNFα).	Single doses of baicalin from 100 mg to 2800 mg have been reported as safe and tolerable. Often given as *Scutellaria baicalensis* (Chinese skulcap) are doses of 200–600 mg one to three times per day	Baicalin is also a cognition support compound due to its neuroprotective and anti-inflammatory effects
Quercetin [40, 41]	NLRP3 inflammasome suppression; stabilizes mast cells; reduces uric acid levels by suppressing xanthine oxidase, antioxidant.	500 mg twice per day	Food sources include: Onions, shallots, green tea, berries, and apples
Genistein [40, 41]	Suppresses NFkB, suppresses mRNA expression level of COX-2, antioxidant.	250 mg twice per day	Commonly used as a phytoestrogen, is a compound found in *Glycine max* (soy)
Naragenin [41]	Suppresses TNF-α, IL-6, TLR4	50 mg bid	Known to inhibit CYP2E1 in the liver—May impact levels of drugs such as cimetidine
Gallic acid [41]	Suppresses NFkB and MAPK	Varies—30 mg twice per day	Berries, grapes, and pomegranate are excellent sources
Kaempferol [40, 41]	Suppresses the release of IL-6, IL-1β, IL-18, and TNF-α; NRF2 activation, inhibits the toll-like receptor 4 (TLR4)	Not commonly found as pure extract—Found in botanical medicines: *Hippophae rhamnoides; Eucalyptus globulus; Bupleurum chinense, Allium cepa, Rhodiola rosea*	Found in capers, saffron, pumpkin, arugula, kale, blueberry, kiwi, gooseberry, and cauliflower, mustard greens, watercress, are good sources

Polyphenol	Mechanism	Dose	Remarks
Ellagic acid [41]	Suppresses PGE-2 and IL-6	500 mg once per day	Found in grapes and pomegranate
Cyanidin [41]	Suppresses PGE2, COX2, and IL-8	Not commonly found as pure cyanidin-3-glucoside but good herbal medicine sources are Grade seed extract (*Vitis vinifera*) and bilberry extract (*Vaccinium myrtillus*), which can both be taken at amounts of 500 mg twice per day or higher	Found in all types of berries commonly eaten, currants, concord grape
Taxifolin [41, 57]	Activates NRF2; suppresses TNF-α, IFN-γ, IL-10, and TLR-4, Neuroinflammation benefits—And reduces production, assembling, and aggregation of amyloid B that can aggregate in neural tissue	50 mg twice per day	Found in *Silybum marianum, Olea europea* but extracts from Siberian larch (*Labrix sibirica*) and higher concentrations are more effective for inflammation control
Chlorogenic acid and isomer cynarin [58]	Suppresses TNF-α, IL-6, IL-8, and IFN-γ. Increases IL-10. Lowers NFkB expression	100 mg twice per day	Eggplant, sunflower seeds, artichoke, coffee, and tea are good sources
Theaflavin-3-gallate [41, 56]	Blocks LPS-induced immune activation (modestly) Reduces NFkB levels Suppresses ERK pathway	Does not appear as a pure extract—Obtained from *Camelia sinensis* tea (oxidized, fermented black tea)	Black tea is an excellent source

Resveratro [40, 41] l	Suppresses IL-1α, IL-6, IL-17, and TNF-α. Inhibits MAPK migration to the nucleus Inhibits COX-2 Neutralizes myeloperoxidase in the arterial environmen	200 mg once per day (higher amounts can be used safely)	Found in many foods including mulberries, lingonberries, red currants, grapes, peanuts, pistachios, bilberries, blueberries, peanuts, and cranberries
Curcumin [40, 41]	Numerous mechanisms and targets Binds to toll-like receptors and reduces NFkB Blocks the NLRP3 inflammasome Activates NRF2 and more production of antioxidant enzymes	500 mg twice per day Should be taken with *Piper nigra* (black pepper) and a fatty food for better absorption Phytosome-bound curcumin (bound to phosphatidylcholine is better absorbed) Liposomal curcumin also has excellent absorption Curcumin nanoparticles have excellent absorption	Turmeric (*Curcuma longa*) is the food that contains curcuminoids (a group of isomers) Foods that have fats such as ghee, butter, or vegetable oils will allow for better absorption Turmeric tea (often combined with other herbs such as ginger (*Zingiber officinale*) are also a source but lack the fatty acid component—So best drunk during or after a meal with some fats
Catechin and related molecules (including epigallocatechin gallate (EGCG)) [54, 56]	Reduces toll-like receptor activation Suppresses IL-1β and TNF-α Reduces matrix metalloproteinase activity Increases superoxide dismutase	100 mg once per day to four time per day	Green and white tea provides catechins. Also apples, spinach, red wine, avocado, onions, and kale

Herbal and mushrooms medicines

Herbal or mushroom extract	Mechanism	Dose	Remarks
Boswellia serrata [52]	Boswellic acid blocks COX2	Encapsulated *Boswellia serrata* 200 mg once per day to three per day	Excellent for joint and soft tissue inflammation
Erigeron breviscapus [48]	Reduces brain inflammation at the vascular level and blocks tau protein and beta-amyloid accumulation in the brain	200 mg once per day or twice per day	Part of the anti-inflammatory effect is also a cognitive boost
Harpagophytum procumbens [53]	Iridoid glycosides that are called harpagosides. Lowers IL-6, TNF-alpha, and COX-2	Encapsulated *Harpagophytum procumbens* 200 mg once per day to three per day	Good for joint and cartilage inflammation
Rosmarinus officinale [49]	Rosmarinic acid, carnosic acid and carnosol reduce inflammasome activation	800 mg once per day or three times per day	Good for neuroinflammation
Cordyceps militaris [50]	β-D-Glcp (1 → 3)-linked reduces inflammatory cytokine levels	200 mg once a day or twice a day	Similar compounds found in other fungi such as *Poria cocos*

Human gut repair and integrity

Recommendation	Mechanism	Dose or behavior	Remarks
Moderate saturated fats [33]	Too much saturated fat may lead to lipopolysaccharide production that is difficult to manage	Eat a variety of foods and consume more than enough dietary fiber along with fatty foods	The issues of saturated fat are compounded in a diet that is low in plant foods and natural antioxidants, low in dietary fiber, and low on sources of substrates of beneficial microflora
Dietary fiber [59, 60]	Sequesters some gut toxins and carcinogens Can bind some fatty acids Promotes positive microflora Fermentation products render short-chain fatty acids that nourish colon epithelium and improve junctions and integrity Can prevent the translocation of bacteria and lipopolysaccharide from gut to portal vein and liver Decreases bowel transit time, thus limiting the persistence of some compounds in the liver	25 to 30 g of fiber per day from diet Dietary fiber supplements can contribute to this such as psyllium husk	Eating whole foods and plant foods can make attaining adequate fiber much easier

Recommendation	Mechanism	Dose or behavior	Remarks
Fermented foods [35, 36]	Provides beneficial microflora and decreases inflammation Healthy microflora competes against more potentially pathogenic bacteria Microbial diversity is associated with less inflammation	At least one serving per day of a live culture food, but multiple food choices that have some cultures effects is better	Being foods, the substrate, the so-called "prebiotics" are present, which help the beneficial microorganisms survive and possible flourish in the gut The fermented foods (yogurts, sauerkraut, kimchi, miso, etc.) have good nutrient density
Probiotic supplements [37, 38]	Provides a strong presence of desired microflora that are gut healing (*Lactobaccilus plantarum, L acidophlius, L rhamnosus, Bifobacteria infantis*) Can change the microbiome, although long term colonization is not guaranteed Some probiotics such as *Bacillus subtilis* helps repair the gut epithelium specifically *Saccharomyces boulardii* can compete against pathogens such as *Clostridium difficile*	The amount varies but can be in the range of 4 billion colony-forming unit (CFU) to 40 billion, or perhaps higher in cases of intensive therapy, per day	Dietary fiber is going to support these microorganisms Some products have oligosaccharides—Prebiotics—To foster growth

Recommendation	Mechanism	Dose or behavior	Remarks
Vitamin A [61]	Support epithelial integrity /tight junctions	Dose depends on diet and other supplementation 5000 IU per day (use beta-carotene in pregnant patients)	Dietary carotenoids can be converted to vitamin A
Vitamin D [61]	Support epithelial integrity /tight junctions	Dose depends on diet and other supplementation 2000 IU per day but may be higher depending on latitude, diet, and individual biochemistry	Serum testing can yield information about D status 50 nmol/L (20 ng/mL) are desirable
Plantago lanceolata (ribwort plantain) [62]	Decrease inflammation, neutralize toxins, promote healing	500 mg dried *Plantago lanceolata* twice per day 5 ml of water–ethanol extract (tincture) twice per day	Similar to dietary fibers but has iridoid glycosides such as aucubin

NOVA classification [25]

NOVA group	Definition	Examples	Health impacts
I	Unprocess, natural foods or minimally processed for edibility but no additions	Fruits, vegetables, meats, oats, rice, pasta yogurt, mushroom, beans, seafood, eggs, milk	Should be the foundation of a diet—Variety and macro- and micronutrients from nutrient-dense options still important
II	Processed culinary ingredients	Oils, fats, honey, maple syrup, butter, coconut oil, vegetable oil, olive oil, sugar	Used as needed along with group 1 foods

NOVA group	Definition	Examples	Health impacts
III	Processed foods	Canned vegetable, pickles, canned fish, fresh baked or artisan breads, salted or cured meat, beef jerky, tomato paste	Can still deliver good nutrients and lower level processing can preserve foods, but group III should not replace group 1
IV	Ultraprocessed foods	Salty snack foods such as potato chips, colas, refined packaged breads such as hot dog buns, candies, cookies, frozen snack food, fast food	Should be limited—Diets high in IV foods will displace other choices and are associated with more cardiovascular disease and cancer

Conclusion

Inflammation is a continuum, and early and self-resolving inflammation and deeper inflammation that becomes self-propagating are closely related phenomena. The impact on the extracellular matrix can be beneficial, such as necessary remodeling and even release and destruction of unwanted molecules (glycated end products, covalent crosslinked molecules, certain toxins that bind to glycoproteins, etc.). It can be costly but necessary, such as stopping invasion by an aggressive or opportunistic (as in certain types of wounds or the immunocompromised patient). It can also become incessant and lead to severe pathologies. Acute inflammatory pathologies are well known and include septic shock and acute organ failure. But chronic inflammatory events in the extracellular matrix in particular lead to permanent damage and disability. Without an intact extracellular matrix, cells simply cannot carry out their intended functions, and the ability of an organ to stay within homeostatic bounds ceases. This is the topic of the next chapter, the advent of fibrosis, and degeneration of the extracellular matrix.

References

1. Arroyo AG, Iruela-Arispe ML. Extracellular matrix, inflammation, and the angiogenic response. Cardiovasc Res. 2010;86(2):226–35.
2. Medicine. The history behind the discovery of toll-like receptors. medicine.yale.edu. 2002. Available from: https://medicine.yale.edu/news/yale-medicine-magazine/article/the-history-behind-the-discovery-of-toll-like-receptors/
3. Roh JS, Sohn DH. Damage-associated molecular patterns in inflammatory diseases. Immune Network. 2018;18(4)
4. Zaru R. Pattern recognition receptors (PRRs): toll-like receptors I British Society for Immunology. www.immunology.org. Available from: https://www.immunology.org/public-information/bitesized-immunology/receptors-molecules/pattern-recognition-receptors-prrs-toll
5. Li D, Wu M. Pattern recognition receptors in health and diseases. Signal Transduct Target Ther. 2021;6(1):1–24.
6. Twarda-Clapa A, Olczak A, Białkowska AM, Koziołkiewicz M. Advanced glycation end-products (AGEs): formation, chemistry, classification, receptors, and diseases related to AGEs. Cells. 2022;11(8):1312.
7. Fulop T, Larbi A, Pawelec G, Khalil A, Cohen AA, Hirokawa K, et al. Immunology of aging: the birth of Inflammaging. Clin Rev Allergy Immunol. 2021;64:1–14.
8. Birch J, Gil J. Senescence and the SASP: many therapeutic avenues. Genes Dev. 2020;34(23–24):1565–76.
9. Ghorbani S, Yong VW. The extracellular matrix as modifier of neuroinflammation and remyelination in multiple sclerosis. Brain. 2021;144(7):1958.
10. Rude KM, Keogh CE, Gareau MG. The role of the gut microbiome in mediating neurotoxic outcomes to PCB exposure. Neurotoxicology. 2019;75:30–40.
11. Prabhu SD, Frangogiannis NG. The biological basis for cardiac repair after myocardial infarction. Circ Res. 2016;119(1):91–112.
12. Genschmer KR, Russell DW, Lal C, Szul T, Bratcher PE, Noerager BD, et al. Activated PMN exosomes: pathogenic entities causing matrix destruction and disease in the lung. Cell. 2019;176(1–2):113–126.e15.
13. Jin Q, Liu T, Qiao Y, Liu D, Yang L, Mao H, et al. Oxidative stress and inflammation in diabetic nephropathy: role of polyphenols. Front Immunol. 2023;14
14. Miguel V, Shaw IW, Kramann R. Metabolism at the crossroads of inflammation and fibrosis in chronic kidney disease. Nat Rev Nephrol. 2024;21
15. Maruyama K, Imanaka-Yoshida K. The pathogenesis of cardiac fibrosis: a review of recent Progress. Int J Mol Sci. 2022;23(5):2617.

16. DiNicolantonio JJ, O'Keefe J. The importance of maintaining a low Omega-6/Omega-3 ratio for reducing the risk of autoimmune diseases, asthma, and allergies. Mo Med. 2021;118(5):453.
17. Minich DM, Brown BI. A review of dietary (Phyto)nutrients for glutathione support. Nutrients. 2019;11(9):2073.
18. Fukai T, Ushio-Fukai M. Superoxide Dismutases: role in redox signaling, vascular function, and diseases. Antioxid Redox Signal. 2011;15(6):1583–606.
19. Kidd P. Th1/Th2 balance: the hypothesis, its limitations, and implications for health and disease. Altern Med Rev. 2003;8(3):223–46.
20. Bulanda S, Janoszka B. Consumption of thermally processed meat containing carcinogenic compounds (polycyclic aromatic hydrocarbons and heterocyclic aromatic amines) versus a risk of some cancers in humans and the possibility of reducing their formation by natural food additives – a literature review. Int J Environ Res Public Health. 2022;19(8):4781.
21. Ng CY, Leong XF, Masbah N, Adam SK, Kamisah Y, Jaarin K. Heated vegetable oils and cardiovascular disease risk factors. Vasc Pharmacol. 2014;61(1):1–9.
22. Cravotto C, Fabiano-Tixier AS, Claux O, Abert-Vian M, Tabasso S, Cravotto G, et al. Towards substitution of hexane as extraction solvent of food products and ingredients with no regrets. Food Secur. 2022;11(21):3412.
23. Penn State Extension. Processing Edible Oils. Penn State Extension. 2013. Available from: https://extension.psu.edu/processing-edible-oils
24. Desilver D. What's on your table? How America's diet has changed over the decades. Pew Research Center. 2016. Available from: https://www.pewresearch.org/short-reads/2016/12/13/whats-on-your-table-how-americas-diet-has-changed-over-the-decades/
25. Nazmi A, Tseng M, Robinson D, Neill D, Walker J. A nutrition education intervention using NOVA is more effective than MyPlate alone: a proof-of-concept randomized controlled trial. Nutrients. 2019;11(12):2965.
26. Martínez Steele E, Baraldi LG, et al. Ultra-processed foods and added sugars in the US diet: evidence from a nationally representative cross-sectional study. BMJ Open. 2016;6(3):e009892.
27. Levy RB, Barata MF, Leite MA, Andrade GC. How and why ultra-processed foods harm human health. Proc Nutr Soc. 2023;83(1):1–8.
28. Monteiro CA, Astrup A. Does the concept of "ultra-processed foods" help inform dietary guidelines, beyond conventional classification systems? YES. Ludwig DS, editor. Am J Clin Nutr. 2022;116(6):1476.
29. de Araújo TP, de Moraes MM, Afonso C, Santos C, Rodrigues SSP. Food processing: comparison of different food classification systems. Nutrients. 2022;14(4):729.
30. Agostino J. Research suggests 73% of food in the U.S. is ultra-processed. Food Tank. 2022. Available from: https://foodtank.com/news/2022/11/database-indicates-u-s-food-supply-is-73-percent-ultra-processed/
31. Mohammad S, Thiemermann C. Role of metabolic Endotoxemia in systemic inflammation and potential interventions. Front Immunol. 2021;11

32. Malesza IJ, Malesza M, Walkowiak J, Mussin N, Walkowiak D, Aringazina R, et al. High-fat, Western-style diet, systemic inflammation, and gut microbiota: a narrative review. Cells. 2021;10(11):3164.
33. González F, Considine RV, Abdelhadi OA, Acton AJ. Saturated fat ingestion promotes lipopolysaccharide-mediated inflammation and insulin resistance in polycystic ovary syndrome. J Clin Endocrinol Metabol. 2018;104(3):934–46.
34. Morrison DJ, Preston T. Formation of short chain fatty acids by the gut microbiota and their impact on human metabolism. Gut Microbes. 2016;7(3):189–200.
35. Cuamatzin-García L, Rodríguez-Rugarcía P, El-Kassis EG, Galicia G, et al. Traditional fermented foods and beverages from around the world and their health benefits. Microorganisms. 2022;10(6):1151.
36. Das G, Paramithiotis S, Sundaram Sivamaruthi B, Wijaya CH, Suharta S, Sanlier N, et al. Traditional fermented foods with anti-aging effect: a concentric review. Food Res Int. 2020;134:109269.
37. Cristofori F, Dargenio VN, Dargenio C, Miniello VL, Barone M, Francavilla R. Anti-inflammatory and immunomodulatory effects of probiotics in gut inflammation: a door to the body. Front Immunol. 2021:12.
38. Virk MS, Virk MA, He Y, Tufail T, Gul M, Qayum A, et al. The anti-inflammatory and curative exponent of probiotics: a comprehensive and authentic ingredient for the sustained functioning of major human organs. Nutrients. 2024;16(4):546.
39. Al Bander Z, Nitert MD, Mousa A, Naderpoor N. The gut microbiota and inflammation: an overview. Int J Environ Res Public Health. 2020;17(20)
40. Yahfoufi N, Alsadi N, Jambi M, Matar C. The immunomodulatory and anti-inflammatory role of polyphenols. Nutrients. 2018;10(11):1618.
41. Rudrapal M, Khairnar SJ, Khan J, Dukhyil AB, Ansari MA, Alomary MN, et al. Dietary polyphenols and their role in oxidative stress-induced human diseases: insights into protective effects, antioxidant potentials and mechanism(s) of action. Front Pharmacol. 2022;13(1)
42. Adak A, Khan MR. An insight into gut microbiota and its functionalities. Cell Mol Life Sci. 2018;76(3):473–93.
43. Fan Y, Pedersen O. Gut microbiota in human metabolic health and disease. Nat Rev Microbiol. 2020;19(1):55.
44. Paynich ML, Jones-Burrage SE, Knight KL. Exopolysaccharide fromBacillus subtilisInduces anti-inflammatory M2 macrophages that prevent T cell–mediated disease. J Immunol. 2017;198(7):2689–98.
45. Deng S, Pei C, Cai K, Huang W, Xiao X, Zhang X, et al. *Lactobacillus acidophilus* and its metabolite ursodeoxycholic acid ameliorate ulcerative colitis by promoting Treg differentiation and inhibiting M1 macrophage polarization. Front Microbiol. 2024;15:1302998.
46. Lu HC, Mackie K. An introduction to the endogenous cannabinoid system. Biol Psychiatry. 2016;79(7):516–25.
47. Anil SM, Peeri H, et al. Medical cannabis activity against inflammation: active compounds and modes of action. Front Pharmacol. 2022;13:13.

48. Jo MJ, Lee JR, Cho IJ, Kim YW, Kim SC. Roots of Erigeron annuus attenuate acute inflammation as mediated with the inhibition of NF- κ B-associated nitric oxide and prostaglandin E2 production. Evid Based Complement Alternat Med. 2013;2013:297427.
49. Borges RS, Ortiz BLS, Pereira ACM, Keita H, Carvalho JCT. Rosmarinus officinalis essential oil: a review of its phytochemistry, anti-inflammatory activity, and mechanisms of action involved. J Ethnopharmacol. 2019;229:29–45.
50. Phull AR, Ahmed M, Park HJ. Cordyceps Militaris as a bio. Microorganisms. 2022;10(2)
51. Jordan PM, van Goethem E, Müller AM, Hemmer K, Gavioli V, Baillif V, et al. The natural combination medicine Traumeel (Tr14) improves resolution of inflammation by promoting the biosynthesis of specialized proresolving mediators. Pharmaceuticals. 2021;14(11):1123.
52. Siddiqui MZ. Boswellia Serrata, a potential Antiinflammatory agent: an overview. Indian J Pharm Sci. 2011;73(3):255–61.
53. Gxaba N, Manganyi MC. The fight against infection and pain: devil's claw (Harpagophytum procumbens) a rich source of anti-inflammatory activity: 2011–2022. Molecules. 2022;27(11):3637.
54. Sartor L, Pezzato E, Garbisa S. (−)Epigallocatechin-3-gallate inhibits leukocyte elastase: potential of the phyto-factor in hindering inflammation, emphysema, and invasion. J Leukoc Biol. 2002;71(1):73–9.
55. Schink A, Neumann J, Leifke AL, Ziegler K, Fröhlich-Nowoisky J, Cremer C, et al. Screening of herbal extracts for TLR2- and TLR4-dependent anti-inflammatory effects. Ojcius DM, editor. PLoS One. 2018;13(10):e0203907.
56. Khan N, Mukhtar H. Tea polyphenols in promotion of human health. Nutrients. 2018;11(1):39.
57. Das A, Baidya R, Chakraborty T, Samanta AK, Roy S. Pharmacological basis and new insights of taxifolin: a comprehensive review. Biomed Pharmacother. 2021;142:112004.
58. Yu Y, Zhang Z, Chang C. Chlorogenic acid intake guidance: sources, health benefits, and safety. Asia Pac J Clin Nutr. 2022;31(4):602–10.
59. Holscher HD. Dietary fiber and prebiotics and the gastrointestinal microbiota. Gut Microbes. 2017;8(2):172–84.
60. Desai MS, Seekatz AM, Koropatkin NM, Kamada N, Hickey CA, Wolter M, et al. A dietary fiber-deprived gut microbiota degrades the colonic mucus barrier and enhances pathogen susceptibility. Cell. 2016;167(5):1339–53.
61. Cantorna MT, Snyder L, Arora J. Vitamin a and vitamin D regulate the microbial complexity, barrier function, and the mucosal immune responses to ensure intestinal homeostasis. Crit Rev Biochem Mol Biol. 2019;54(2):184–92.
62. Zhang S, Hu J, Sun Y, Tan H, Yin J, Geng F, et al. Review of structure and bioactivity of the Plantago (Plantaginaceae) polysaccharides. Food Chem X. 2021;12:100158.

Fibrosis and Extracellular Matrix Degeneration: Examples of Extracellular Matrix Involvement and Treatment

10

Having examined the way in which inflammation can self-propagate, intensify, and degrade the extracellular matrix, we now turn to examining the consequences of this destruction. The aftermath of past or ongoing inflammation is not simply an ability of the ECM to repair itself as quickly as structures—proteoglycans, fibrillar proteins, polysaccharides—are being torn down. In fact, the opposite seems to be the case. The hyperproliferation of collagen is a recurrent finding in various ECM settings, an overly exuberant response to injury, while initially an adaptive response, ultimately becomes a maladaptive one.

In this chapter, we will examine examples of this process, which has some form of fibrosis as a consistent feature and leads to the breakdown of ECM architecture. The term is used deliberately here as the structure of the ECM is laid down for specific purposes. When that structure begins to change, it has an immediate effect on the cells that are bound up with that ECM. These effects involve changes to the mechanotransduction signaling that has an impact on cell growth, proliferation, and migration. The various growth factors stored in vesicles (exosomes, and microvesicles) associated with small leucine-rich proteoglycans may be available at different levels, as may apoptotic bodies. The dispersion of arterial blood with oxygen and nutrients to cells may be constrained by fibrosis. The removal of CO_2-rich blood and various toxins (including metabolic byproducts) could be constrained.

F. Smith, *The Extracellular Matrix in Health and Disease*,
https://doi.org/10.1007/978-3-031-94465-9_10

Many of these effects of fibrosis and ECM degradation can be seen in the loss of specific microstructures necessary for function of a tissue or organ.

Pathways to Fibrosis

The common cellular pathway is the activation of myofibroblasts. The cytokine transforming growth factor beta will activate connective tissue growth factor, which will cause differentiation of fibroblasts to myofibroblasts that become active secretors of collagen and fibronectin [1–4]. The precise mechanisms of fibrosis vary between tissues, with fibrotic genes activated in the kidney, or stellate cells converting to myofibroblasts in the liver, or also involving actin in muscle fibrosis. Fibroblasts differ between organs and can even differ within an organ with different layers or zones of tissues having their own fibroblast types.

When tissues are injured and inflammatory mediators are present, there is more activation of matrix metalloproteinase (MMP). These powerful enzymes can degrade collagen and are part of normal remodeling. These are normally suppressed by tissue inhibitors of metalloproteinases (TIMP). [5] Excessive matrix degradation by MMP, which can happen when injury and inflammation are prolonged or excessive, will activate transformation of fibroblasts to myofibroblasts. This leads to fibrotic deposition (Fig. 10.1). This can develop in a tissue-specific way. Another matrix degrading enzyme is the series of ADAM enzymes (a disintegrin and metalloproteinase), which are secreted by fibroblasts, epithelial cells, and some immune cells. Excessive metalloproteinase release goes beyond a normal remodeling function and leads to a counter-reaction of excessive collagen deposition—fibrosis.

Fibroblast growth factors (FGFs) can also spur a fibrotic response. One type of FGF is FGF23. This is produced by osteoblasts and osteoclasts and is involved in phosphate and vitamin D function. But in abnormal amounts, as would occur in chronic kidney disease, FGF23 can cause myocardial fibrosis with thickening of the left ventricle [6–8]. Conversely, the angiotensin II

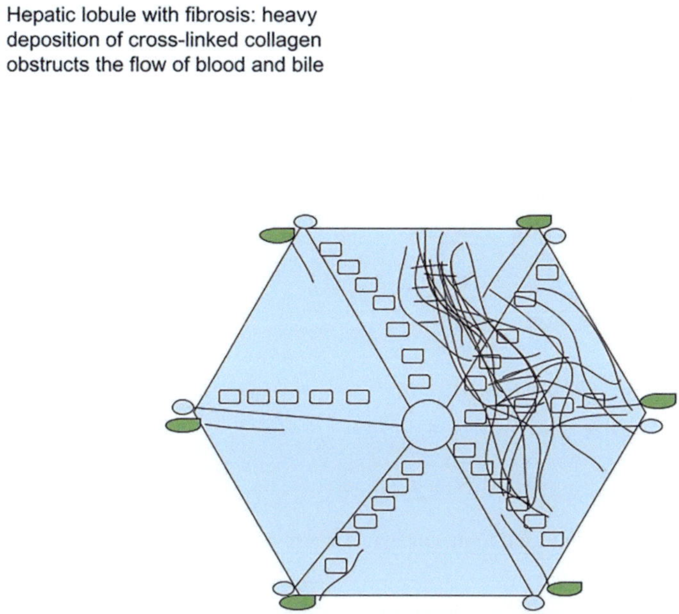

Fig. 10.1 Hepatic fibrosis

that arises from increased renin secretion from the kidneys in heart failure can itself damage the kidneys [9].The elevated intraglomerular pressure caused by renin, while it may allow the kidney to continue to function in states of low cardiac output, eventually leads to fibrosis.

Injurious Events That Activate Fibrotic Pathways

Inflammation can lead to fibrosis as stated above. Inflammatory activators such as tumor necrosis factor alpha (TNF-a), interleukin 6, and 8 (IL6, IL8), and monocyte chemoattractant protein will all lead to tissue damage and that in turn ignites innate immune responses. As outlined in the previous chapter, components of damaged cells—such as histones and mitochondrial DNA—and matrix (such as hyaluronic acid fragments) will be

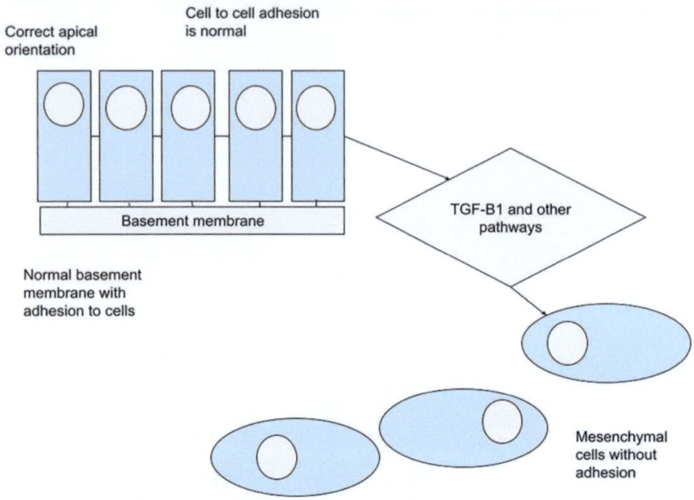

Fig. 10.2 Epithelial-to-mesenchymal transition

taken up by pattern recognition receptors. These include Toll-like receptors, NOD receptors, and the inflammasomes inside of macrophages [10–12]. This will provoke more inflammation. This process can also induce epithelial-to-mesenchymal transition in tissues, which is a pro-fibrotic change (Fig. 10.2).

Increased NF-kB (nuclear factor kappa-light-chain-enhancer of activated B cells) will lead to TGF-beta. Combined with angiotensin II, it can provoke fibrosis. c-Jun N-terminal kinases (Jun) can activate pro-fibrotic genes. TGF can also activate the Janus Kinase (JAK)-Signal Transducer and Activator of Transcription (STAT) pathways within cells, which also has a transcription effect on increasing fibrosis.

Oxidative Stress

Aerobic activity in the cell mitochondria will create oxygen radicals. The mitochondria is the site of oxidative phosphorylation [13]. Some electrons, especially in the presence of high oxygen and increased activity, leak out of the mitochondrial inner membrane. Superoxide ($O2^{\bullet-}$) is the most common by-product. Superoxide can create hydrogen peroxide (H2O2) and the hydroperoxyl radical (HO2•). When superoxide combines with nitric oxide (NO•), which is ubiquitous in the body, especially the vascular endothelium, it will form peroxynitrite (ONOO−). Another species that can derive from superoxide is the hydroxyl radicals (•OH) under certain conditions (Fig. 10.3).

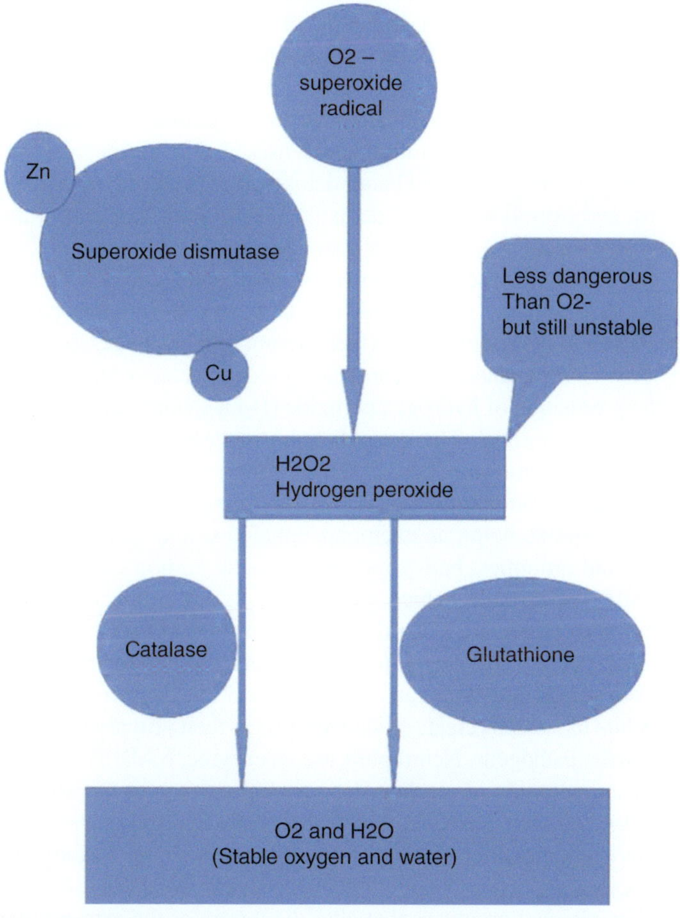

Fig. 10.3 Superoxide dismutase

Oxidative stress is also present as a result of various oxidases in the body and can certainly damage the ECM [14]. The best known are the mixed function oxidases known as the cytochrome system. Cytochrome P450, which is a superfamily with many constituent isozymes, is a first step in detoxification of xenobiotics and some internal toxins [15]. The actual purpose of P450 is to oxidize a compound so that it can be rapidly conjugated to a so-called phase 2 molecule, such as glutathione or glucuronic acid, rendering it water soluble and hopefully harmless. Some form very reactive intermediaries during phase 1 or P450 oxidation, and some of these oxidative compounds damage surrounding cell structures (including membranes of cells and organelle) before they can be conjugated. This can lead to a propagation reaction where an unpaired electron is passed from molecule to molecule. The cell has multiple defenses against this process, but the nature of the compound being detoxified, its kinetics, nutritional status, and overall burden on detoxification systems can impact the net oxidative stress arising from detoxification.

Quinone reductases enzymes will convert endogenous or dietary quinones (including some alkaloids that have uses in naturopathic medicine) to hydroquinones, which are not oxidative stressors. But in some circumstances this can lead to more oxidative stress, such as the production of hydrogen peroxide (H_2O_2), which can turn into the hydroxyl radical. The detoxification process for quinones can also produce semi-quinones, which can foster oxidative stress.

Oxidative compounds can also occur from various toxins, with cigarette smoke being an exemplar. Inhaled smoke has hydroquinones and quinones, heavy metals, aromatic carbon compounds, and nitrogen dioxide, which can react with other tobacco smoke compounds (there are several thousand of them) to form reactive oxygen species [16]. Air pollution contains particulate matter and organic compounds that can also create reactive oxygen species.

White blood cells create oxidative stress as their primary means of destroying pathogens. Neutrophils use an enzyme, NADPH oxidase, to make superoxide, an electron-deficient form of oxygen. Superoxide leads to hydrogen peroxide, which will create hydroxyl radicals. In chronic inflammatory states, neutrophils, as well as eosinophils, monocytes, and macrophages, will create superoxide [17].

Physiological processes that alter the terrain of the extracellular matrix can also induce oxidative stress. For instance, in the accumulation of triglyceride in the hepatocytes, which can be non-alcoholic fatty liver disease or alcoholic fatty liver disease, the fatty acids can begin to oxidize. Whatever naturally present antioxidants including tocopherols are present, they are overwhelmed by the sheer amount of fatty acids. This reactive can self-propagate. Mitochondria will attempt to process some fatty acids via beta-oxidative, but this again leads to stress on the mitochondria. Mitochondria begin to dysfunction, and the liver cells rely more on glycolysis, which in turn adds to oxidative stress. Initial damage leads to increased stiffening of the ECM in the liver, which can in time activate a fibrotic positive feedback loop through the release and activation of several growth factors, primarily transforming growth factor (TGF-β) [18–20].

Fibroaging

This term refers to the process of increasing extracellular matrix stiffness during the aging process (Fig. 10.4). As previously described, in conditions of accelerated biological aging, such as high levels of advanced glycation end products, and an inflammatory phenotype, the stiffening of ECM is more pronounced. This is due to Lysyl oxidases, and some nonenzymatic covalent fusions of colla-

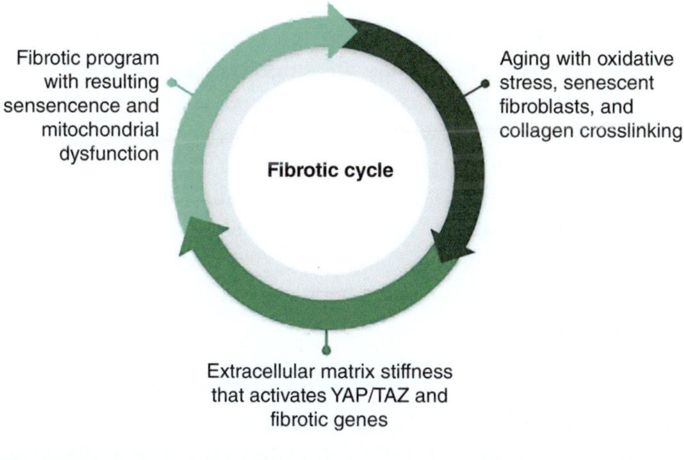

Fig. 10.4 Stiffness and fibrosis

gen molecules together. This stiffening in itself can activate TGF-B, leading to fibroblast differentiation into myofibroblasts. This leads to more fibrosis, more stiffening, and more TGF-B production [21].

Consequences of Fibrosis

Fibrosis will induce a progress process, starting with impaired of circulation and a rapid upregulation of inflammation, and more fibrosis. The consequences of fibrosis vary depending on the type of organ. In the kidney, tubulointerstitial fibrosis and glomerulosclerosis result. In the liver, ultimately cirrhosis will destroy function. In the lungs, the elasticity, recoil, and normal ventilation of the lung are reduced. Muscles that are fibrotic lose their normal contractility. Splenic fibrosis leads to loss of the vital lymphatic tissue. Central nervous and peripheral nervous [22] system fibrosis can result from injury, and this has a large effect on healing or permanent loss of function. Joints can lose their cartilage function due to eventual fibrosis [23].

Treatment Measures

Dietary Considerations

The dietary practices discussed in the preceding chapter of this textbook are useful in creating an antifibrotic terrain in the body. Foods that are rich in antioxidant and antioxidant enzyme supporting nutrients will assist with reducing oxidative stress and inflammation. The microbiota in the human gut can be pro-inflammatory when the composition of species becomes abnormal, and this can be prevented with dietary fiber and fermented foods.

Methylation

High circulating levels of homocysteine have been reported for patients with hepatic fibrosis. Homeocystenia is associated with poor function of the methylation enzymes. Although some forms of fibrosis are characterized by excessive methylation of DNA, a lack of methylation may also accelerate some forms [24].

S-adenosylmethionine, created from methionine, is the primary methyl donor in the body. The compound methyltetrahydrofolate (5-MTHF or sometimes known as "L methylfolate") is needed to maintain adequate methionine levels. Human metabolism can create 5-MTHF from dietary folate but it is an inefficient conversion. Dietary folate is converted to dihydrofolate (DHF) by the enzyme dihydrofolate reductase (DHFR), an enzyme that can further convert DHF to tetrahydrofolate (THF). Ultimately, the enzyme methylenetetrahydrofolate reductase will convert products of DHF to the truly active form of folate (B9), which can be used to convert homocysteine back to methionine. Dietary folic acid must be converted to folate via DHFR. This conversion of folic acid to folate is not efficient.

Genetic polymorphism of the MTHFR activity are common [25–27]. Some are likely to be clinically significant and others occasionally so. About 35 very serious polymorphisms of MTHFR are known but are fortunately rare. About nine polymorphisms are more common and vary in significance. The two most common are C677T and A1298C—the numbering system alluding to the gene they are located in. Some people are heterozygous for polymorphism and can operate their MTHFR system almost as well as average. Testing for these variants yields precise information, which needs to be interpreted in the light of the true impact on the individual—in other words, simply having a polymorphism does not result in automatic 5-MTHF issues.

Generally, the following configurations are of clinical significance.

Polymorphism	Percentage loss of MTHFR function in heterozygotes (approximately)	Percentage loss of MTHFR function homozygotes (approximately)
MTHFR C677T	40%	70%
MTHFR A1298C	20%	40%
MTHFR C677T & MTHFR A1298C heterozygous	No homozygous form as this is a heterozygous genotype	50%

Vitamin B6 is needed for conversion of THF to a form that can be acted on by MTHFR. Vitamin B2 is needed for the actual MTHFR enzyme. Vitamin B12 works with 5-MTHF in the conversion of homocysteine to methionine. Specific sources are given in a table below, but in general: whole grains, meats, brewer yeast, fish, eggs, leafy greens, and nuts. Folate in particular can come from legumes, leafy greens, liver, okra, and some sea vegetables. Natural folates tend to be in a polyglutamate form that must be hydrolyzed to make the monoglutamate form in the gut in order for absorption to occur.

Foods fortified with folic acid may have limited value. FA has to be converted to DHF using the same enzyme that is used to turn dietary folate to DHF— the enzyme listed above—dihydrofolate reductase. Excessive supplemented FA can saturate this enzyme, leading to the buildup of unmetabolized folic acid in the body that can have neurologic effects and can potentially mask a deficiency of vitamin B12.

Individuals with confirmed or suspected MTHFR polymorphism of consequence should simply supplement with the active form L-methylfolate, also known as 5-MTHF, as well as a diet with forms of natural folate (even though conversion to 5-MTHF will be poor, there will still be some and what dietary contributions can be made are probably from foods rich in the other cofactors such as B2, B6, and B12).

Antioxidant Enzymes and Nutritional Support

Cells and the extracellular matrix are protected from oxidative stress by free-floating antioxidants, both plant compounds and nutrients vitamin C. The antioxidant enzymes that process reactive oxygen species are mainly intracellular (although enzymes such as superoxide dismutase are found in the ECM). The primary antioxidant enzymes intracellularly are superoxide dismutase, catalase, and glutathione synthase and reductase. Even though these are within cells, their importance in preventing fibrotic reactions in the ECM is via preventing the cellular necrotic events that can trigger pattern recognition receptors. That pathway will lead to inflammatory reactions with attendant protease release and increased oxidative stress in the ECM. This can be part of normal remodeling or can become destructive enough to release excessive collagen production and crosslinking. Fibrotic reactions are driven by transforming growth factor beta (TGFbeta), which activates Smad proteins. These proteins have several effects, but as transducers of TGFbeta, they can lead to exuberant collagen production by fibroblasts.

Superoxide dismutase (SOD) catalyzes [28] the reaction where superoxide is turned into hydrogen peroxide. This is still a potential free radical as it can become the hydroxyl radical, so it must be further acted on by protective enzymes. Catalase can turn hydrogen peroxide into water and stable oxygen. Another fate of hydrogen peroxide is for glutathione peroxidase to create water and glutathione disulfide. The latter can be recycled into usable glutathione by glutathione reductase. SOD has copper, zinc, and manganese types. Catalase has an iron-containing heme group. Glutathione peroxidase needs selenium, and glutathione reductase needs riboflavin (B2), vitamin E, and vitamin C [29].

Antifibrotic Plant Extracts

Punica granatum (Pomegranate)

Pomegranate extracts have been found to inhibit toxin-induced hepatic fibrosis [30, 31]. A rich source of polyphenols such as ellagic acid and punicic acid, it has also been found to inhibit cardiac fibrosis. These compounds not only directly absorb oxidative compounds, they activate antioxidant enzymes via the NRF2 pathways and inhibit NFkB. Moreover, pomegranate extracts inhibit mitogen-activated protein kinase (MAPK), which is overactivated under conditions of inflammation and can lead to fibrosis.

Astragalus membranaceus (Astragalus)

This plant has a long history in traditional Chinese medicine and other systems. It is known to be an immune upregulator. One of its compounds, Astragaloside IV, a tetracyclic triterpenoid saponin, has antifibrotic effects, including protection against pulmonary fibrosis [32, 33]. Formonentin, another *Astragalus* compound, can inhibit cardiac fibrosis. *Astragalus* polysaccharides can inhibit peritoneal fibrosis. Calycosin, an isoflavone (also found in *Trifolium pratense* (red clover)), is protected against hepatic fibrosis. This is done through the inhibition of inflammatory pathways and reductions in TGF-beta, like many other plant antifibrotics. It also protects mitochondria from ischemic injury, which might be particularly important in protecting against peritoneal fibrosis.

Rosmarinis officinalis (Rosemary)

Rosemary is a fragrant shrub that is widely used in cooking. It is rich in terpenes that form the basis of essential oils. These include alpha and beta pinene, cineole, and β-caryophyllene. It also contains Rosmarinic acid, a caffeic acid ester [33, 34]. This compound has antifibrotic effects that include NRF2 activation and MAPK inhibition (much as *Astragalus*), as well as activation peroxisomal proliferator-activated receptor gamma (PPARγ). It can reduce the effects of TGFbeta and the Wnt pathway (a signaling pathway that can be overactive in fibrosis).

Rosmarinic acid is also found in *Melissa officinalis* (lemon balm), *Ocimum basilicum* (holy basil), Prunella vulgaris (heal all), *Salvia miltiorrhiza* (red safe), *Glechoma hederacea* (creeping charlie), *Coleus forskohlii* (coleus), and many other plants.

Silybum marianum (Milk Thistle)

This plant is well known to reduce inflammation in the liver due to oxidative stress and protect against hepatic fibrosis. The flavonolignans, collectively known as silymarin, include silibinin, silydianin, and silichristin. These compounds increase glutathione levels in cells and absorb free radicals. Silymarin may also reduce excessive matrix metalloproteinase activity in the ECM. It can reduce stiffness in livers that are already fibrotic [35–37].

Berberine

The alkaloid berberine, found in plants such as *Mahona (Berberis) aquafolia* (Oregon grape), *Hydrastis canadensis* (Goldenseal), and *Coptis chinensis* (Goldenthread), has antifibrotic effects. It can suppress epithelial-to-mesenchymal transition, a step toward extensive fibrosis in an organ [38].

Eleutherococcus senticosus (Siberian Ginseng)

This plant is one of the first to be studied in the twentieth century as having adaptogen properties. It does increase endurance and tolerance of chronic stress. The acanthopanaxosides are triterpene saponins and have effects on cortisol levels and white blood cell levels. This herb also can help polarize human macrophages to the M2 polarization. This is an anti-inflammatory macrophage role, with less matrix metalloproteinase release [39].

Artemisia annua (Chinese Wormwood)

Artemisia is a genus with many medicinal species in it around the world. A compound found in it—artemisinin, a sesquiterpene lactone—has been made into a highly effective antimalarial drug. This compound also has been found in an animal model to block cardiac fibrotic hyperplasia due to the suppression of MAPK and ERK pathways. An extract of *Artemisia argyi* (a similar species) was found in a mouse model to inhibit hepatic fibrosis [40].

Cordyceps sinensis

Caterpillar fungus is known to increase stamina and immune function, but it also has antifibrotic effects [41]. It may have an application in renal fibrosis.

Scutellarin is a flavonoid from plants such as *Scutellaria baicalensis* (Chinese skullcap). It is used as a cognitive support herb but it may also decrease the factors, leading to pulmonary fibrosis [42, 43].

Antioxidant systems

Enzyme	Function	Cofactors	Food sources
Superoxide dismutase [28, 44]	Converts peroxide radical to H_2O_2	Zinc, copper, and manganese SOD	Mn: Brazil nuts, shellfish, brown rice, leafy greens Zn: Meat, seafood, nuts, legumes, sweet potatoes, avocados Cu:Avocado, lima beans, seafoods, liver, cocoa, peanuts, pistachios (note: Copper should not overpower zinc in the diet)
Catalase [44]	Converts H_2O_2 to H_2O and O_2	Iron in a heme structure	Fe: Meats, leafy greens, legumes, iron-fortified foods
Glutathione peroxidase [29, 44]	Converts H_2O_2 to H_2O	Selenium	Se: Poultry, eggs, and whole grains, pork, beef, mushrooms
Glutathione reductase [29, 44]	Reduces used glutathione back to reduced glutathione disulfide	Riboflavin (B2)	Liver, whole grains, tempeh, fish, almonds, meat, shiitake mushrooms, anchovies

Plant extracts and fibrosis

Plant	Mechanism	Dose	Remarks
Punica granatum [30]	Polyphenols such as ellagic acid and punicic acid inhibit (MAPK) and are antioxidants	Pomegranate extract 400 mg two times per day	Eating the food is beneficial. There are also pomegranate-concentrated juices on the market that are rich in the polyphenol compounds

Plant	Mechanism	Dose	Remarks
Astragalus membranaceus (Astragalus) [45, 46]	Astagaloside IV, formononetin, calycosin, and polysaccharides reduce inflammation, TGF-activation	Two 500 mg capsules two times a day Tincture (water and ethanol extract) 3 ml two times per day (or higher if needed to 5 ml two times per day)	A very versatile anti-fibrotic. This plant has a very long use in traditional Chinese medicine, and is also an adaptogen and immune tonic
Rosmarinic acid (found in a variety of plants including *Rosmarinus officinalis*—Rosemary) [33, 34]	Activation of NRF-2, decreases TGF-beta	Depends on herbal source *Rosemarnius officianlis* (rosemary) 500 mg two times per day	Has been shown to reduce fibrosis in rheumatoid arthritis
Silybum marianum and its flavonolignan (silymarin including silibinin, silychristin, silydianin) [36, 37, 47]	Increases glutathione levels in cell, and balances activating of matrix metalloproteinases	Standardized extract of *Silybum marianum* with 80% flavonolignans 300 mg two times per day	Is protective to liver cells and kidney cells and reduces inflammation as well as preventing excessive ECM degradation that can lead to fibrotic reactions

Plant	Mechanism	Dose	Remarks
Berberine (from *Hydrastis canadensis, Coptis chinensis, Mahonia aquifolium, Mahonia vulgaris, Berberis aristata* (which is more typically used as a *source* of berberine) [48]	Suppresses epithelial to mesenchymal transition Some anti-inflammatory effects	Berberine 500 mg twice per day	Generally safe although prolonged and excessive consumption could lead to oxidative stress in the liver due to berberine being an isoquinoline alkaloid (the quinone aspect of the molecule requires adequate antioxidant enzymes in the liver)
Eleutherococcus senticosus (Siberian ginseng) [39]	Acathopanaxosides lead to polarization of macrophages to M2, which reduces metalloproteinase activity	500 mg twice per day	Can be used in tincture and in traditional Chinese medicine, is boiled (decoction) with other herbs, an efficient method for extracting polysaccharides
Artemisia annua (Chinese wormwood) [40]	Suppression of MAPK and ERK by artemisinin	Artemisinin 100 mg 1× per day Tincture (water–ethanol extract) of *Aremisia annua* 2 ml twice per day	Artemisinin and modified forms (such as the drug artemether) are very effective against some strains of malaria Related species such as *Artemisia absinthium* can have higher amounts of alpha and beta thujone that can pose toxicity to the nervous system

Plant	Mechanism	Dose	Remarks
Cordyceps sinensis [41]	Reduces epithelial-to-mesenchymal transition	200 mg *Cordyceps sinesis* in capsules twice per day	Has anti-fatigue, immune, and chemopreventive uses
Scutellarin from *Scutellaria baicalensis* [42, 43]	Inhibits NF-κB/NLRP3-mediated epithelial–mesenchymal transition	Tincture (water ethanol extract) 3 ml twice per day	*Scutellaria lateriflora*—Used as a nervine and sedative, also has this flavonoid

References

1. Hinz B. The extracellular matrix and transforming growth factor-β1: tale of a strained relationship. Matrix Biol. 2015;47(47):54–65.
2. Wynn TA, Vannella KM. Macrophages in tissue repair, regeneration, and fibrosis. Immunity. 2016;44(3):450–62.
3. Wynn TA, Ramalingam TR. Mechanisms of fibrosis: therapeutic translation for fibrotic disease. Nat Med. 2012;18(7):1028–40.
4. Antar SA, Ashour NA, Marawan ME, Al-Karmalawy AA. Fibrosis: types, effects, markers, mechanisms for disease progression, and its relation with oxidative stress, immunity, and inflammation. Int J Mol Sci. 2023;24(4):4004.
5. Brew K, Nagase H. The tissue inhibitors of metalloproteinases (TIMPs): an ancient family with structural and functional diversity. Biochim et Biophys Acta (BBA) Mol Cell Res. 2010;1803(1):55–71.
6. Isakova T. Fibroblast growth factor 23 and risks of mortality and end-stage renal disease in patients with chronic kidney disease. JAMA. 2011;305(23):2432.
7. Morita H, Hoshiga M. Fibroblast growth factors in cardiovascular disease. J Atheroscler Thromb. 2024;31(11):1496–511.
8. Maruyama K, Imanaka-Yoshida K. The pathogenesis of cardiac fibrosis: a review of recent Progress. Int J Mol Sci. 2022;23(5):2617.
9. Xu Z, Li W, Han J, Zou C, Huang W, Yu W, et al. Angiotensin II induces kidney inflammatory injury and fibrosis through binding to myeloid differentiation protein-2 (MD2). Sci Rep. 2017;7(1)
10. Huebener P, Schwabe RF. Regulation of wound healing and organ fibrosis by toll-like receptors. Biochim Biophys Acta (BBA) – Mol Basis Dis. 2013;1832(7):1005–17.
11. Bale S, Verma P, Varga J, Bhattacharyya S. Extracellular matrix-derived damage-associated molecular patterns (DAMP): implications in systemic sclerosis and fibrosis. J Invest Dermatol. 2023;143(10):1877–85.

12. Alyaseer AAA, de Lima MHS, Braga TT. The role of NLRP3 Inflammasome activation in the epithelial to mesenchymal transition process during the fibrosis. Front Immunol. 2020;11
13. Murphy MP. How mitochondria produce reactive oxygen species. Biochem J. 2008;417(1):1–13.
14. Rees MD, Kennett EC, Whitelock JM, Davies MJ. Oxidative damage to extracellular matrix and its role in human pathologies. Free Radic Biol Med. 2008;44(12):1973–2001.
15. Cichoż-Lach H. Oxidative stress as a crucial factor in liver diseases. World J Gastroenterol. 2014;20(25):8082.
16. Caliri AW, Tommasi S, Besaratinia A. Relationships among smoking, oxidative stress, inflammation, macromolecular damage, and cancer. Mutat Res Rev. 2021;787:108365.
17. Winterbourn CC, Kettle AJ, Hampton MB. Reactive oxygen species and neutrophil function. Annu Rev Biochem. 2016;85(1):765–92.
18. Caligiuri A, Gentilini A, Pastore M, Gitto S, Marra F. Cellular and molecular mechanisms underlying liver fibrosis regression. Cells. 2021;10(10):2759.
19. Lambrecht J, Mannaerts I, Leo. The role of miRNAs in stress-responsive hepatic stellate cells during liver fibrosis. Front Physiol. 2015;6
20. Schwabe RF, Tabas I, Pajvani UB. Mechanisms of fibrosis development in nonalcoholic Steatohepatitis. Gastroenterology. 2020;158(7):1913.
21. Selman M, Pardo A. Fibroageing: an ageing pathological feature driven by dysregulated extracellular matrix-cell mechanobiology. Ageing Res Rev. 2021;70:101393.
22. Mietto BS, Mostacada K, Martinez AMB. Neurotrauma and inflammation: CNS and PNS responses. Mediat Inflamm. 2015;2015:1–14.
23. Fu B, Shen J, Zou X, Sun N, Zhang Z, Liu Z, et al. Matrix stiffening promotes chondrocyte senescence and the osteoarthritis development through downregulating HDAC3. Bone Research. 2024;12(1):32.
24. Pineda-Tenor D, Gómez-Moreno AZ, Sánchez-Ruano JJ, Artaza-Varasa T, Virseda-Berdices A, Fernández-Rodríguez A, et al. *MTHFR* rs1801133 polymorphism is associated with liver fibrosis progression in chronic hepatitis C: a retrospective study. Front Med. 2020;7:582666.
25. Raghubeer S, Matsha TE. Methylenetetrahydrofolate (MTHFR), the one-carbon cycle, and cardiovascular risks. Nutrients. 2021;13(12):4562.
26. de Carvalho SCR, Muniz MTC, Siqueira MDV, Siqueira ERF, Gomes AV, Silva KA, et al. Plasmatic higher levels of homocysteine in non-alcoholic fatty liver disease (NAFLD). Nutr J. 2013;12(1)
27. Hu Y, Liu J, Dong X, Xu Y, Leng S, Wang G. Clinical study of serum homocysteine and non-alcoholic fatty liver disease in Euglycemic patients. Med Sci Monit. 2016;22:4146–51.
28. Fukai T, Ushio-Fukai M. Superoxide Dismutases: role in redox signaling, vascular function, and diseases. Antioxid Redox Signal. 2011;15(6):1583–606.

29. Minich DM, Brown BI. A review of dietary (Phyto)nutrients for glutathione support. Nutrients. 2019;11(9):2073.
30. Maphetu N, Unuofin JO, Masuku NP, Olisah C, Lebelo SL. Medicinal uses, pharmacological activities, phytochemistry, and the molecular mechanisms of Punica granatum L. (pomegranate) plant extracts: a review. Biomed Pharmacother. 2022;153:113256.
31. Mannino F, Imbesi C, Bitto A, Minutoli L, Squadrito F, D'Angelo T, et al. Anti-oxidant and anti-inflammatory effects of ellagic and punicic acid in an in vitro model of cardiac fibrosis. Biomed Pharmacother. 2023;162:114666.
32. Song L, Zhang W, Tang S, Luo S, Xiong P, Liu J, et al. Natural products in traditional Chinese medicine: molecular mechanisms and therapeutic targets of renal fibrosis and state-of-the-art drug delivery systems. Biomed Pharmacother. 2023;170:116039.
33. Boo YC. Therapeutic potential and mechanisms of Rosmarinic acid and the extracts of Lamiaceae plants for the treatment of fibrosis of various organs. Antioxidants. 2024;13(2):146.
34. Borges RS, Ortiz BLS, Pereira ACM, Keita H, Carvalho JCT. Rosmarinus officinalis essential oil: a review of its phytochemistry, anti-inflammatory activity, and mechanisms of action involved. J Ethnopharmacol. 2019;229:29–45.
35. Choi S, Ham S, Lee YI, Kim J, Lee WJ, Lee JH. Silibinin downregulates types I and III collagen expression via suppression of the mTOR signaling pathway. Int J Mol Sci. 2023;24(18):14386.
36. Aghemo A, Alekseeva OP, Angelico F, Bakulin IG, Bakulina NV, Bordin D, et al. Role of silymarin as antioxidant in clinical management of chronic liver diseases: a narrative review. Ann Med. 2022;54(1):1548–60.
37. Gillessen A, Angelico F, Chen J, Lu L, Lucena MI, Fu Q, et al. Silymarin for treating toxic liver disease: international consensus recommendations. Gastro Hep Adv. 2022;1(5):882–93.
38. Avila-Carrasco L, Majano PL, Sánchez-Tomero JA, Selgas R, López-Cabrera M, Aguilera A, et al. Natural plants compounds as modulators of epithelial-to-mesenchymal transition. Front Pharmacol. 2019;10
39. Jin L, Schmiech M, El Gaafary M, Zhang X, Syrovets T, Simmet T. A comparative study on root and bark extracts of Eleutherococcus senticosus and their effects on human macrophages. Phytomedicine. 2020;68:153181.
40. Erdenebileg S, Kim M, Nam Y, Cha KH, Le TT, Jung SH, et al. Artemisia argyi ethanol extract ameliorates nonalcoholic steatohepatitis-induced liver fibrosis by modulating gut microbiota and hepatic signaling. J Ethnopharmacol. 2024;333:118415.
41. Zhang Y, Li K, Zhang C, Liao H, Li R. Research progress of Cordyceps sinensis and its fermented mycelium products on ameliorating renal fibrosis by reducing epithelial-to-mesenchymal transition. J Inflamm Res. 2023;16:2817–30.

42. Peng L, Wen L, Shi QF, Gao F, Huang B, Meng J, et al. Scutellarin ameliorates pulmonary fibrosis through inhibiting NF-κB/NLRP3-mediated epithelial–mesenchymal transition and inflammation. Cell Death Dis. 2020;11(11):978.
43. Nie S, Zhang S, Wu R, Zhao Y, Wang Y, Wang X, et al. Scutellarin: pharmacological effects and therapeutic mechanisms in chronic diseases. Front Pharmacol. 2024;15
44. FDA. Vitamins VITAMIN WHAT IT DOES WHERE IT IS FOUND DAILY VALUE* Biotin. 2021. Available from: https://www.accessdata.fda.gov/scripts/interactivenutritionfactslabel/assets/InteractiveNFL_Vitamins&MineralsChart_October2021.pdf
45. Zhu Y, Chai Y, Xiao G, et al. Astragalus and its formulas as a therapeutic option for fibrotic diseases: pharmacology and mechanisms. Front Pharmacol. 2022:13.
46. Tan YQ, Chen HW, Li J. Astragaloside IV: an effective drug for the treatment of cardiovascular diseases. Drug Des Dev Ther. 2020;14:3731–46.
47. Terzi F, Ciftci MK. Protective effect of silymarin on tacrolimus-induced kidney and liver toxicity. BMC Complement Med Ther. 2022;22(1):331.
48. Cely-Veloza W, Kato MJ, Coy-Barrera E. Quinolizidine-type alkaloids: Chemodiversity, occurrence, and bioactivity. ACS Omega. 2023;8(31):27862–93.

Organ Failure: Examples of Extracellular Matrix Involvement and Treatment

11

The extracellular matrix is distinctly altered in chronic organ diseases that are moving toward what is clinically termed organ failure. This is also true of chronic degenerative states that are not organ specific but pertain to distinct tissue—such as ECM changes in a synovial joint with very advanced arthritic changes. Due to the dynamic interplay between ECM and cells, the changes to the matrix in chronic disease are both cause and effect. Problems that affect cells across an organ will lead to reactions in the ECM. For example, destruction of hepatocytes due to an autoimmune condition will provoke inflammation that ultimately disrupts the local ECM. If that disruption leads to fibrosis, those results will negatively impact the function of any remaining hepatocytes. If myocytes die due to a myocardial infarction, the resulting inflammatory remodeling will involve the matrix and lead to excessive collagen deposition.

Conversely, matrix abnormalities can impact the cell [1]. When the ECM becomes stiff, as in the case of fibrotic reactions, excessive collagen and fibronectin deposition, abnormal covalent collagen crosslinking, accumulation of advanced glycation end products, etc., it alters the behavior of cells. Mechanotransduction effects that operate via integrin and various second messenger systems, as well as direct signals sent via the cytoskeleton, can change gene transcription in the cell. Cell proliferation and migra-

F. Smith, *The Extracellular Matrix in Health and Disease*,
https://doi.org/10.1007/978-3-031-94465-9_11

tion are influenced by the ECM. Likewise, the mitochondria of cells are influenced by ECM properties.

A stiff matrix not only dysregulates many cell behaviors; it can ultimately confer a senescent phenotype on the cell [2]. This can be observed to have less productive activity, weaker mitochondria, and, in some cases, a pro-inflammatory disposition. Cells are intimately and vitally bound up with their surrounding ECM. The term Anoikis was created in the 1990s by Frisch and Francis, who discovered that peeling the ECM away from cells, breaking the integrin attachments, leads to programmed cell death [3]. Some cells learn to bypass the Anoikis program, and this is a hallmark of many cancer cells.

The precise nature of ECM breakdown of course depends on the microstructure of that tissue-specific matrix. It is reflected in alternations in the architecture of the organ or local tissue type. Excessive density of renal extracellular matrix will impair the normal filtration process. A fibrotic spleen will be less efficient at filtering the blood and moving senescent red blood cells (red pulp) or providing immune scavenging and responses via lymph tissue (white pulp). A fibrotic liver will show plenty of type I collagen in the zones around hepatocytes and grossly, cross-cutting collagen structures that broadly interrupt canalicular and vascular flow.

The clinical management of organ failure, chronic disease, and any situation and advanced tissue atrophy is a challenge. Naturopathic medicine has much to offer in these situations with treatments that both support organ function and natural sources of molecules that can often induce higher levels of function. Without question, conventional medical approaches are paramount in organ failure. The fact that cells and their structures have broken down means that very precise interventions will be needed. External support to override maladaptive responses and keep the body in some degree of homeostasis is needed—as any heart failure patient using sodium-depleting diuretics to prevent pulmonary edema or any advanced emphysema patient using home oxygen can attest. Moreover, advanced pathologies can often progress and destabilize the entire organism very rapidly. Conventional therapies that can be implemented and altered quickly, and that work assertively are well suited to these situations.

It can reasonably be asked if there is any clinical utility in working on the ECM when it is at this level of dysfunction. At lower levels of dysfunction, various treatments to support, protect, and heal the ECM are helpful. But what about the instances where the ECM is already degraded? The answer is partly that certain therapies can offset the loss of requisite ECM functions for cellular viability. In advanced organ disease, the continued ECM degradation may accelerate loss of that organ or tissue's cells due to the lack of ECM support [4]. For the remaining cells, the broken ECM can also induce certain changes that accelerate dysfunction.

Two prominent issues are the lack of normal autophagy and the expression of senescent phenotypes. These two phenomena go hand in hand and are discussed below. In summary, autophagy is the necessary breakdown of unneeded cellular waste, particularly proteins that have exceeded their useful life span. A diseased ECM will impair normal autophagy. Likewise, the stiff, oxidized, and overly dense ECM will induce sensent behaviors in cells. Adhesion complexes built around the transcellular protein integrin literally sense stiffness. This is transduced into the nuclear activity of YAP and TAZ proteins, which leads to more cell proliferation, a possible cancer risk [5]. A lack of stiffness allows for the release of focal adhesion kinase (FAK) molecules in a soluble form leading to the activation of mTORC2. This is an inhibitor of mTORC1, and when the latter is inhibited, the autophagy program can execute including expression of APG genes.

Senescence and stiff matrix conditions extend to nearby stem cells, which become less capable of fulfilling their replacement role. Naturopathic therapies can help induce these necessary functions, even if the underlying state of affairs is chronic, and quite often progressively worse.

Autophagy and Mitophagy

Cells have a mechanism for clearing out defective structures that not only permits replacement but working copies of proteins but prevents the cell from becoming literally cluttered with waste. Autophagy is the name for a vacuole formation that occurs in the cell [6–8]. This is supplemented by some cell membrane (secretory) forms of autophagy. In the primary autophagy process, the gene ATG1 (AuTophaGy related 1) is expressed, which leads to the formation of an autophagic vesicle (there are multiple ATG subtypes with a similar function with 1 being common). This will grow and then fuse with a lysosome, which has powerful digestive enzymes, kept away from the rest of the cell. This complex will engulf and digest structures that are drawn to the lysosome through protein chaperones. It should be noted that a separate pathway for clearing molecular waste in the cell is the proteasome pathway. The proteasome is a special protein that degrades other proteins that are marked for destruction by the attachment of multiple ubiquitin proteins.

ATG1 activation occurs as mTOR (mammalian target of rapamycin) is suppressed, specifically, the mTORC1 protein. Generally, mTOR is a bridge between signals such as insulin, and states such as well-fed or fasting, and the regulation of metabolism, cell proliferation, and autophagy. The fasting state causes intracellular rise in a class of proteins called Sirtuins (SIRT), and SIRT1 in particular is an upregulator of ATG1, and therefore autophagy. The caloric restricted state also raises the levels of a cellular energy indicating protein, MAPK (5' AMP-activated protein kinase), which is also a pro-autophagy signal (Fig. 11.1).

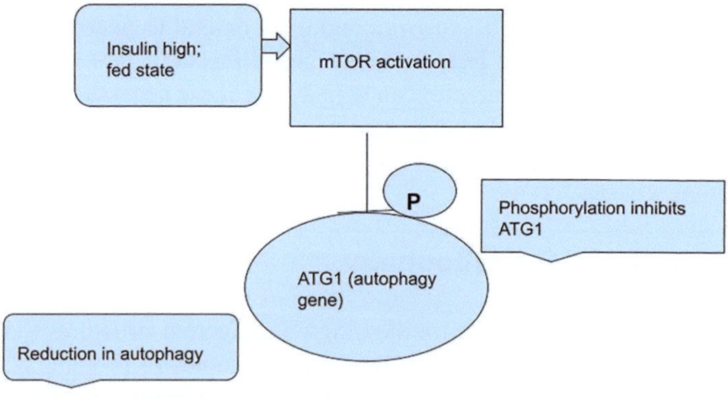

Fig. 11.1 ATG1 inhibition-fed state

Stiffness means more YAP and TAZ persistence, and cell proliferation. Cell-to-cell adhesion and extracellular matrix binding to the cell, such as decorin, kringle5, and collagen VI, will suppress mTOR and increase ATG expression. Decorin is a prominent autophagy inducer and can also induce mitophagy, whereby damaged, low-output mitochondria can be subjected to autophagic destruction. This is beneficial for any cell, and especially so for cells with high energetic needs, such as cardiomyocytes.

Senolytics

Cells age into a senescent phenotype as they accrue damage to genes, mitochondria, membranes, and organelles [9, 10]. Apoptosis of senescent cells is ideal, and this generally succeeds in keeping their population in check, in younger organisms. With age comes a higher standing level of senescent cells, which can lead to disease. A strong presence of senescent cells can push someone into a senescence-associated secretory phenotype (SASP) [11]. This individual will have a state of "sterile inflammation" with more activation of pattern recognition receptors, and higher levels of cytokines that drive inflammation (such as IL-6). Another feature is disordered extracellular matrix, with overactivation of proteases and consequent reactive fibrosis. This has been discussed in previous chapters, and there are excellent naturopathic therapies for dampening the effects of this inflammation and getting a person out of the SASP state.

Another therapeutic approach, which is the subject of intense research, is to create therapies that reduce the number of senescent cells in the body [10]. That is, they reduce the population of senescent cells so that the standing levels of such cells are more like a younger organism. Both synthetic and natural agents are under investigation for this property, and some natural options are discussed below.

An aged extracellular matrix is senescence inducing. Cells are less able to resist conversation to a senescent phenotype in a fibrotic and deformed matrix. This becomes a self-reinforcing cycle of sensent behaving cells fostered by a dysfunctional ECM, which leads to more damage to the ECM and a less viable environment for cells. Even though, in advanced diseases, some organ damage is permanent, and even progressive, effort can still be directed to removing senescent cells and creating an ECM that is not permissive.

Organ-Specific Consequences of Degenerated ECM and Opportunities for Naturopathic Support

Cardiac Hypertrophy and Cardiac Dilatation

Heart failure has demonstrable changes to the ECM [12, 13]. This is both as a consequence of previous events and ongoing pathology, and is a driver of progressive deterioration of heart function. After a myocardial infarction, there is often a zone of myocardial necrosis. During the repair and remodeling process, some fibrous tissue will be laid down to stabilize the area, which is under constant strain due to the normal filling and pumping actions of the heart. That scar tissue will later lead to a less resilient myocardium. The collagen in cardiac scar tissue is the normal type I and III collagen, but also contains type V collagen, which is normally present in the dermal–epidermal junction, but not the heart. This leads to a stiffer heart and pathology progresses from there.

As a heart enters progressive phases of heart failure, it can become a pressure overloaded and hypertrophic heart, or a dilated and weak heart. Both types of progression show extensive ECM remodeling. In the case of hypertrophy, the production of collagen is ongoing and can lead to thickening and more stiffness. Clearly, this will have an adverse effect on autophagy and mitophagy, leading to the persistence of essence cells and an abnormally high population of dysfunctional mitochondria.

Initial heart failure can lead to this thickening with transition of cells, particularly macrophages, to myofibroblasts that secrete abundant collagen. This will transition in time to a more inflammatory state where MMP and ADAM enzymes begin to destroy ECM of the heart. This leads of course to various matrikines—

proteins of the matrix—and their fragments attaching themselves to pattern recognition receptors. This includes Toll-like receptors and intro macrophage inflammasomes. This leads to more inflammation and destruction. There are many variants of heart failure with degrees of diastolic or systolic, muscular or electrical, dysfunction but this evolution of ECM function corresponds to a common clinical pathway.

In the early stages of heart failure with diminished left ventricular output due to some previous injury, the stiffening and hypertrophy of the heart and blood vessels lead to poor diastolic filling and increased peripheral resistance. In this state, medications such as angiotensin conversion enzyme blockers or angiotensin receptor antagonists provide great relief. The relaxation of peripheral vessels and reduction in sympathetic inputs into the heart allow for better diastolic filling and more cardiac output, including improved ejection fraction due to decreased peripheral resistance. As the disease progresses, these medicines still help, but the degenerative changes in the heart gather momentum, and in time, keeping the heart, kidneys, lungs, brain, and other organs in balance becomes impossible. This is not a shortcoming of routine medical regimen for heart failure, which have expanded life expectancy for heart failure patients and quality of life. It is indicative, however, of the necessity to adapt therapy to changes in terrain, including ECM dissolution.

Renal Fibrosis

Chronic kidney disease can develop from many causes, including autoimmune nephritis, hypersensitivity reactions, the effects of acute or chronic heart failure on the kidney, and various systemic and metabolic diseases such as cirrhosis of the liver. A common pathway for these conditions is an increase in inflammation and levels of NFkB, with a resulting exuberant production of extracellular matrix [14, 15]. Overwhelming amounts of angiotensin II in the kidney can activate these fibrotic changes as well. TGFbeta is converted into an active form and sets in motion myofibroblast activity. Continued thickening of ECM will have immediate effects of decreasing glomerular filtration rate. Over time, it will lead to glomerulosclerosis and tubulointerstitial fibrosis.

A cardiorenal axis has long been recognized and is increasingly understood [16–18]. Poor perfusion of the kidney due to a low cardiac ejection fraction will lead to failure and renal acidosis but for the activation of the renin–angiotensin–aldosterone system (RAAS) from the kidney. This will lead to sodium retention and volume expansion and increase postglomerular pressure and intraglomerular pressure, allowing the organ to continue to function. Chronic kidney disease leads to electrolyte imbalances and RAAS activation, which can impact cardiac function. Alterations in serum electrolytes have negative effects on the heart, such as hyperkalemia. Excessive blood pressure will damage the heart (and overtime lead to more kidney fibrosis).

Splenic Fibrosis and Inflammation

Of several splenic diseases, one that speaks to the themes of this chapter is heart-related splenic changes. The term "cardio-splenic" axis has been proposed to describe the cycle of pathological changes in these two organs and how those changes can reinforce each other's progression [19–21]. Alternated hemodynamics and inflammatory cytokines released into the circulation in heart failure cause a reactive remodeling in the spleen. This leads to enlarged white pulp (the lymphatic core of the spleen) with the release of inflammatory mediators that accelerate inflammation and fibrosis in the heart.

Lung Fibrosis and Oxygen Issues

The ECM changes in pulmonary diseases, with increased stiffness in the asthmatic patient leading to more reactivity to stimuli. This stiffness is partly due to collagen crosslinking that occurs due to ongoing inflammation. In pulmonary fibrosis, uncontrolled collagen deposition will render an extremely stiff lung that has ventilation issues due to lack of recoil [22]. In emphysema, destruction of the ECM renders it inflexible (not only stiff locally but too stiff to expand properly) with poor ventilation to perfusion ratio due to loss of alveolar walls. In the case of emphysema and chronic obstructive lung disease, there will be hypoxia and extra stress on the right ventricle [23]. Many patients with COPD and fibrosis have pulmonary hypertension as a result of remodeling of tissues in the lung.

Hepatic Failure and ECM

The development of chronic liver disease is one of toxin exposure, mitochondrial damage, cellular necrosis, inflammation, and excessive stellate cell conversion to myofibroblasts [24].

Once the excessive collagen deposition has taken place, the blood from the portal system can no longer flow properly through the liver. This leads to impaired input of nutrients from the gut and less ability to filter out toxins [25–27]. Aside from the circulatory deficit, reductions of viable hepatocytes add to the problem. Portal hypertension can lead to ascites, and gut toxins can do their worst, without a proper detoxification system in place to intercept them [28].

Sarcopenia and ECM

In aging muscle, there are alternations in the ECM characterized by excessive collagen deposition. There is also a lack of fibronectin in these muscles, leading to a lack of connections to integrin. The organization of collagen changes, to move from a very ordered array of collagen fibers to a more erratic one. This will crowd out myosatellite cells, which are stem cells that are needed for muscle replacement. This leads to muscle degeneration. The disordered ECM to mitochondria connections due to local of focal adhesion kinases leads to mitochondrial dysfunction [29, 30].

CNS ECM Collapse and Implications

The variety of neurodegenerative conditions, their etiology and treatment, is beyond the scope of this chapter. But with regards to the ECM and neurodegenerative conditions, there are some frequent findings. Perineural nets are specialized ECM structures rich in chondroitin sulfate proteoglycans. They stabilize the dendritic connections and balance inhibitory and excitatory signals in the brain. Their absence leads to a loss of effective brain function [30–32].

Overproduction of hyaluronic acid in the early plaques of neurodegenerative conditions, apparently in the earlier evolution of these lesions. Overproduction and deposition of hyaluronic acid can suppress oligodendrocyte precursor cells (OPC). This is highly detrimental, as OPC are needed for myelin production, and myelin is crucial to the proper transmission of electrical signals along the nerve [32].

Many of these aberrations are due to excessive inflammation and oxidative stress, which can activate microglial response and provoke more inflammation, and damage. These lesions in the brain are to some extent a response to injury. This also includes astrocyte expansion and glial scar formation, which are features of inflammation and trauma. This can include strokes, infections, or physical trauma.

Treatment

Two axes of treatment are explored in this chapter. One is focused on attempting to rehabilitate the autophagic and senolytic functions of the tissues. The other is focused on biochemical support that is directed at more extracellular matrix features of the organ's declines. As noted above, these ECM states are both cause and consequence of many chronic diseases. This focus is in keeping with the purpose of this textbook and is not meant to discount the many other helpful approaches to chronic illness, including a broader use of naturopathic therapies, acupuncture, and to the great benefit of patients with extreme pathologies, and conventional approaches.

Hormesis as an Autophagy Inducer

Inducing autophagy genes, increasing Sestrins, and changing the balance of mTORC2 to mTORC1 can foster this activity. As noted, this is important in aging and aged extracellular matrices, which themselves will inhibit autophagy and mitophagy. The behaviors and plant extracts that can induce autophagy appear to do so in ways that have hormetic features. That is, they present challenging effects of small magnitude (mild stressors) to elicit an adaptive response by the organism and its cells (Fig. 11.2).

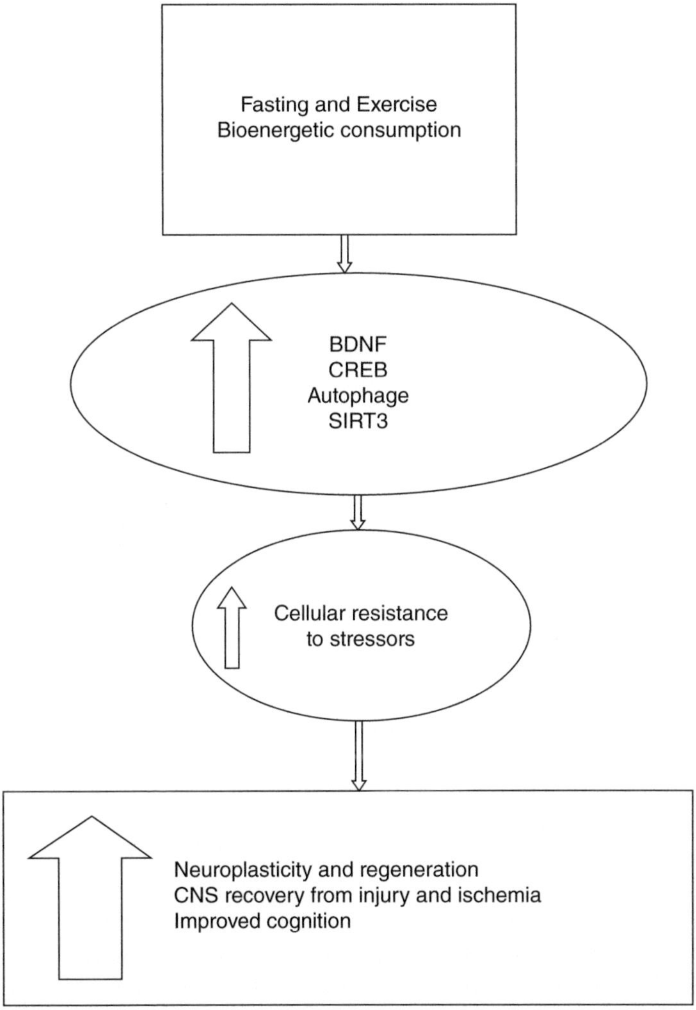

Fig. 11.2 Hormetic and fasting inputs CNS example

Caloric Restriction

Intermittent fasting pertains to fasts of designated lengths that are interrupted by feedbacking periods. For example, a patient who does a 24-h fast (water only), once a week, could be said to do intermittent fasting. How long is it necessary to initiate autophagic responses? It may be as short as 16 h. One pattern is to eat within 8-h windows during the day to allow for more optimal autophagic periods. This eating period can be shrunk to 6 h or 4 h. Another method is scheduling one or two fasting days per week (24 h each fasting day). Fasting beyond 24 h is an ancient practice. Fasts beyond 3 days should be medically supervised. Diabetes and those with more advanced health issues should be medically supervised.

Caloric restriction does increase Sestrin levels and autophagy [33, 34]. Aside from fasting, limiting the calories of regular meals may have a pro-autophagy effect. Isocaloric twice-a-day eating, so the regular and energy-balanced caloric intake but limited to two feedings, is suggested to induce autophagy in animal models, and this may translate to humans.

Quercetin is an inducer of autophagy. By activating the Forkhead box O (FOXO) gene, quercetin and block MTORC1 upregulated autophagy. This polyphenol has other important effects on inflammation and even the tumor microenvironment [35].

Unlike the other examples listed here of autophagy induction, berberine protects against excessive autophagy, which is a possible outcome of ischemic damage to the heart. After myocardial injury, repair and remodeling processes activate to address the damaged myocardium. Too much autophagy in heart muscle cells that might have remained viable leads to their apoptosis [36].

Astragalus membranaceus promotes autophagy. This plant contains triterpenoid saponins, flavonoids, and polysaccharides. *Astragalus*-driven autophagy can protect mitochondria in the heart under conditions of stress from the chemotherapeutic agent doxorubicin. It may also reduce skin aging due to UV photodamage [37].

Spermidine is a naturally produced polyamine in the body that is an autophagy inducer. Fasting will increase spermidine levels. Foods such as wheat germ, soybeans, chickpeas, green peas, aged cheddar cheese, mushrooms, and chicken liver are some of the good sources [38].

Hydrotherapy

Exposure to cold and heat has been found to enhance autophagy. The naturopathic therapies considered as "hydrotherapy" could have pro-autophagy actions. For example, constitutional hydrotherapy treatment involves alternating hot and cold applications to the chest and abdomen, and back. This improves circulation, digestion, and elimination, but could also provide a positive stimulus to autophagy. Likewise, sauna therapy could have their supportive role [39].

Senolytics

Some compounds, including those from plants, can induce senolysis—the apoptosis of dysfunctional senescent cells. These aging cells have defective mitochondria and other damaged organelles. In the extracellular matrix, senescent fibroblasts do not produce the proteins that are needed for a healthy ECM. In organs generally, the senescent cell population can swell as that organ becomes progressively dysfunctional. While senolytic inputs can lower that population, they will not regenerate the organ itself. But the shift toward a healthy senolytic activity is beneficial, and in naturopathic medicine, we are trying to support the body through multiple mechanisms and reduce the stressors on the body where possible.

Some of the better researched senolytics are quercetin and fisetin. [40, 41] These compounds can induce apoptosis by encouraging pro-apoptosis signals to overpower suppressors in the cell. They also suppress inflammation and reduce the kind of cytokines that senescent cells secrete.

Fisetin is a yellow flavonoid found in onions, strawberries, and persimmons. It can inhibit Bcl-2-type genes and have an apoptosis-promoting effect. Quercetin has a similar impact on apoptosis of a senescent cell and on inflammation. This anti-senescent phenotype effect is found across multiple organs and is also seen to some extent with other polyphenols. These effects are also found in muscle, cartilage, and bone, which of course have aging-related deterioration.

Examples of Organ-Supporting Treatments

In naturopathic medicine, there are hundreds of remedies, nutritional, and physical medicine options that can help support the function of the body. In the section below, we will examine some that are exemplary in helping beleaguered organs and tissues continue to function as best they can. These treatments can encourage some organ repair and healing, especially in conjunction with a broad effort to address the determining and required factors of health, remove obstacles to healing including external stressors and toxins, and treat the whole person. The organ systems influence each other, which is by definition their role to play in the body. But upon further examination, many organs have very direct linkages that are continuing to be elucidated. For example, the spleen and heart have a connection whereby excessive inflammatory production by the white pulp (lymph) of the spleen can increase the inflammatory damage occurring in some kinds of chronic heart disease. The gut and the brain have an "axis" that has been well described, with communication via the vagus (CN X) nerve and various compounds that emerge from the gut such as serotonin. There are examples in traditional medicine systems of these kinds of influences—with the five-element process in acupuncture and several East Asian medical systems being a common one. In strictly biomedical terms, the physiological and metabolic dependencies that organs have on one another create fixed relationships between them. The study of specific crosstalk between organs can yield insight into how to alleviate distress in them. For example, cardiorenal syndrome is well described, as is the heart–lung relationship in chronic disease.

Ginkgo biloba: Vascular and Brain

Ginkgo or the "maidenhair tree" is an ancient species of tree that almost went extinct. It is widely planted now and even thrives on the boulevards of large cities in spite of the pollution. Ginkgo contains triterpene glycosides and ginkoflavoneglycones. A standardized extract of Ginkgo (GBE) is quite consistent in composition and used in many studies. EGb761 is a German product that became the basis for GBE. It has 24% flavone glycosides and 6% terpenes (compounds such as ginkgolides).

Ginkgo has protective effects on the brain and vascular system. It reduces oxidative stress in vascular tissues and protects the vascular endothelium [42, 43]. It can cause some vasodilation in muscular arteries. As a pretreatment, it has hormetic effects in that myocardial cells exposed to Ginkgo have better tolerance of ischemia. It is also useful in peripheral vascular disease, including popliteal artery stenosis.

Ginkgo has brain protective effects, with less deposition of amyloid in animal models of dementia. It has a protective effect on the hippocampus. In human trials, there have been some benefits for patients with dementia. The use of *Ginkgo biloba* for those with cerebrovascular disease is helpful because Ginkgo appears to rehabilitate the vascular endothelium, which ought to improve blood flow to the brain [44].

Ginkgo is protective to another highly vascular tissue—the kidney. It can help with diabetic nephropathy and reduce oxidative stress and ferroptosis—iron-catalyzed oxidative destruction of kidney cells. It can reduce extracellular matrix accumulation in the kidney as well as transition of renal cells to mesenchyme. Ginkgo can protect the kidney against vancomycin toxicity. Vancomycin is a powerful antibiotic reserved for difficult-to-treat infections, most notably, *Clostridium difficile* infections of the gut [45].

Silybum marianum: Liver and Kidney

Milk thistle in a plant with historical uses as a liver tonic. It does have some bitter qualities and can act as a digestive tonic. *Silybum marianum* contains flavonoids that are collectively referred to as Silymarin, a portmanteau name from the genus and species. Silymarin has flavonoids such as silibinin, silydianin, and silychristin. These compounds have been investigated for their biological and clinical effects for decades. Silymarin is strongly protective of the liver. In an animal model, it can even protect the liver against powerful experimental toxins such as carbon tetrachloride.

Silmyarin is a very powerful antioxidant and can stabilize the cell and organelle membranes of the liver [46, 47]. This is useful for toxins that become so after being metabolized as well as those that are toxic as soon as they are absorbed from the gut. SIlmyarin has been found to increase glutathione levels in the cell, possibly due to a glutathione-sparing effect. It has some stimulating effect on protein synthesis [48].

In human trials, it has been found to lower transaminases in patients with chronic viral infection or alcoholic cirrhosis, and liver biopsy specimens take on a more normal appearance. It is not established that Silymarin increases life expectancy in a disease such as cirrhosis. A more recent line of inquiry for the use of Silymarin is to treat nonalcoholic fatty liver disease (NAFLD). This is a very common condition, where the liver has a high amount of triglyceride. About a third of the US adult population and possibly 10% of the pediatric population have NAFLD. When the liver has this amount of triglyceride, the oxidation of those fatty acids, and damage to mitochondria, can result in nonalcoholic hepatosteatosis (NASH). This can progress to cirrhosis. Siymarin can lower gamma-glutamyl transferase (GGT) and indicator of NAFLD severity.

In chronic states of liver inflammation, eventually there is fibroblast to myofibroblast conversion. Stellate cells in the liver will elaborate collagen to the point where it becomes obstructive. Silymarin has been found to decrease liver stiffness in patients who had some hepatic fibrosis due to previous viral hepatitis. This indicates that as a de-stiffening agent it might help rehabilitate extracellular matrix to some degree in the liver.

Milk thistle is most often given in a standardized extract form, which is 80% silymarin. In some countries, such as Slovakia or Germany, intravenous silymarin is administered after some poisonings, such as injection of *Amanita phalloides,* the death cap mushroom [49].

Silymarin has been found to have some protective effect on the kidney against toxins and perhaps the heart as well. While this is less researched, it is plausible given the known mechanisms of the flavonoids [50].

Crataegus oxycantha: Heart

Hawthrone is a widely used treatment for heart disease. It is rich in flavonoids such as vitexin and in polyphenols. It has been studied clinically, and while it will not erase chronic damage due to previous events, it does help the heart to contract more efficiently. It is, for those with heart failure, particularly left ventricular heart failure with diminished ejection fraction, positively inotropic and negatively chronotropic. In human trials, it has been found, on Doppler ultrasound, to increase ejection fraction [51]. Hawthorne seems to relax the arteries and increase blood flow to the myocardium. Perhaps the most significant function of Hawthorne is the ability to rehabilitate the vascular endothelium [52]. When this inner lining of the artery is damaged, it dysfunctions, synthesizing less nitric oxide, which leads to vessel tightening. Localized inflammation allows for more damage to occur when oxidized LDL is deposited in the intima. Moreover, the powerful antioxidants of Hawthorne are helpful to protect the endothelial glycocalyx, an ECM-like projection into the vascular flow from the endothelial cells. This area has proteoglycans and heparin sulfate and has the ability to regulate what kinds of molecules come into direct contact with the endothelium.

Patients given Hawthorne can report better quality of life, better exercise tolerance, improved abilities at daily activities, and fewer symptoms of congestive heart failure. It may also protect the heart against ischemia reperfusion injury, so it is likely to have pretreatment and proactive effects.

Crocus sativa: Brain

Saffron is a treasured and often very expensive spice. It is made from the stigma and styles of the plant and is produced in Iran, India, Greece, Spain, and Morocco. This plant has remarkable effects on brain health and function. It contains crocins (carotenoids), flavonoids, and monoterepenes (crocusatins). It has antidepressant and antianxiety effects. Being a powerful antioxidant, it may reduce chronic, low-grade neuroinflammation, which can exacerbate mood disorders [53–55]. It reduces oligodendrocyte destruction, which is helpful in diseases such as Parkinsons and multiple sclerosis. It has been shown to reduce amyloid plaques, although this is more preventive than remediating dementia. It may protect neurons from the effects of injury-preventing apoptosis in neurons that could still be viable. While the experimental and (limited) human trials with saffron do not indicate that it will reverse many of these degenerative conditions, the ability of this plant to normalize neural tissue is a reason to consider giving it. The strong antioxidant effects will decrease neuroinflammation, which helps prevent reactionary depositions of brain ECM (higher in chondroitin sulfate as opposed to collagen as found in other ECMs in the body).

Vinpocetine

This semisynthetic product is made from *Vinca minor (*periwinkle). It is derived from the alkaloid vincamine in the plant. It can assist with impaired cerebral circulation overall and has been found in human clinical trials to protect against neuronal damage due to ischemia [56, 57]. Used post stroke, it can reduce damage. It targets cyclic nucleotide phosphodiesterase 1 (PDE1). It can prevent overactivation of the sodium channel after cellular injury, which prevents cell death. It also inhibits NFkB. This substance reduces inflammation in blood vessels and is neuroprotective. It may help prevent post-myocardial infarction damage but this is not clear yet. It does reduce the inflammation in hearts that are undergoing remodeling due to high angiotensin levels. It is not safe in pregnancy as it is teratogenic and lethal. Vinca alkaloids inhibit mitosis, which is why high doses of them are used to treat some cancers. Although vinpocetine might not have the amount of suppression of mitosis (the alkaloids inhibit spindle formation during prophase and metaphase) for an adult, this substance is not to be used in pregnancy or for infants or young children.

Hippophae rhamnoides: **Heart**

Sea buckthorn is an edible plant originally found in Eurasia but cultivated around the world, including North America. The juice is sold as a nutrient-dense food. Sea buckthorn has a panoply of compounds in it. There are flavonolignans, including silibinin (as does *Silybum marianum*—milk thistle). There are other flavonoids such as isorhamnetin and quercetin, as well as terpenes such as limonene and sesquiterpenes and phenylpropanoids. There are other phenolic compounds such as catechin, epicatechin, gallocatechin, and epigallocatechin. Sea buckthorn is a comprehensive blend of some of the most important phenolic compounds including flavonoids.

Sea buckthorn is strongly anti-inflammatory across many tissues of the body [58]. It is cardioprotective and even has some antimicrobial effects. In the sense that ECM degradation due to aging, diet, hyperglycemia, and persistent oxidative stress causes an inflammatory phenotype to emerge, sea buckthorn could be useful as part of a plan to change that inflammatory state.

Panax ginseng: **Heart**

Ginseng has a very long history of use in traditional East Asian medical systems as a whole-person tonic. It contains triterpenoid saponins known as ginsenosides. The plant has anti-fatigue and immune-supporting functions. It is classified as an adaptogen, which means it can improve human endurance and resistance to stress, without a direct stimulatory action. It improves blood flow to the heart via eNOS, creating more nitric oxide and thus blood flow [59]. It also protects the heart against reperfusion damage. It may also support mitochondria [60]. Ginseng can moderate the activity of matrix metalloproteinases, preventing overly asserting remodeling or even degradation of the ECM [61]. It also has broad anti-inflammatory properties [62].

Nigela sativa: Brain

Black cumin is a neuroprotective herb, with traditional uses for healing wounds. It has powerful antioxidant functions, inhibiting NFkB, and MMP activity. It improves acetylcholine levels in the brain. It blocks cyclooxygenase. It is protective of brain tissue in general [63–66].This herb seems appropriate for assisting patients who have aging and damage to the extracellular matrix of the brain, which can lead to microglial activation and neuroinflammation. This is particularly well indicated with someone suffering from cognitive impairment, which has attendant changes to the ECM, including collapse of perineural nets.

Colchicum autumnale: Heart and Kidney

The autumn crocus contains the alkaloid colchicine. This was used traditionally for the treatment of gout. It appears to reduce the amount of inflammation in the toes due to the rupture of phagocytic cells that had encountered uric acid crystals in the gout patient. Colchicine is used in medicine again, with new uses for the heart and kidney. It reduces fibrosis in the diabetic kidney [67, 68]. In patients treated with colchicine post-myocardial infarction, it reduces the excess deposition of ECM proteins and reduces the formation of neutrophil extracellular traps. A defensive action of neutrophils during infection is to create webs of DNA and proteins to bind up pathogens. These are also formed after acute myocardial infarction. This can accentuate the post-MI damage by increasing inflammation, platelet aggregation, and oxidative stress [69, 70]. Colchicine is a prescription drug, and the form of this alkaloid that is likely to be used in acute/ hospital medicine (Fig. 11.3). In a chronic sense or other conditions, the tincture of *Colchicum autumnale* could have benefits.

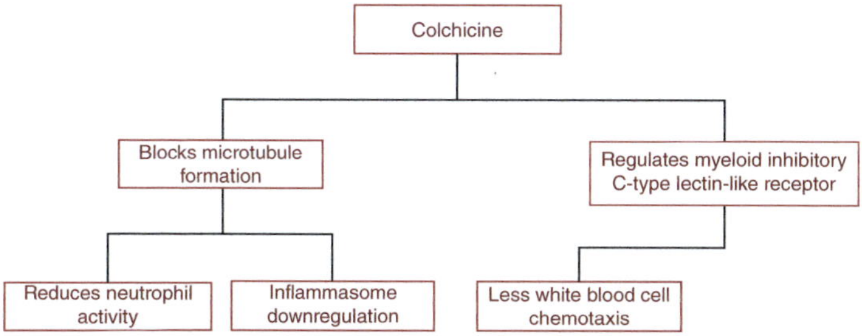

Fig. 11.3 Colchicine

Pro-autophagy and senolytic treatments

Treatment	Mechanism	Dose	Remarks
Quercetin [35]	Activates the Forkhead box O (FOXO) gene, quercetin and block MTORC1 and upregulated autophagy	500 mg per day.	Found in onions, grapes, apples, kale, broccoli
Berberine [36]	Stimulates autophagy via ERK1/2 pathway. Protects against excessive autophagy.	500 mg twice a day	Also found in herbs such as *Mahonia* (*Berberis*) *aquafolia*
Astragalus membranaceus [37]	Triterpenoid saponins influence the AMPK/mTOR pathway.	500 mg twice a day or three times a day; tincture (water—Ethanol extract) 3 ml twice a day or three times a day	Some preparations have additional astragalosides added to them
Caloric restriction [34]	Cellular energy needs increase leading to higher sestrin levels and autophagy.	Eating restricted to 8 hours out of the day. Two fasting days per week	There are many fasting and caloric-restrictive plans. The patient's goals, physiological state, comorbidities, and motivation have to be taken into consideration

Treatment	Mechanism	Dose	Remarks
Spermidine [38]	Inhibition of acetyl acetyltransferases	10 mg twice a day or three times a day	Spermidine is found in foods such as wheat germ, soybeans, chickpeas, green peas, aged cheddar cheese, mushrooms, and chicken liver
Fisetin [71]	A powerful antioxidant, nearly identical to quercetin—Precise mechanism unclear	10 mg once a day	Found in pistachios, almonds, grapes, and like quercetin, in onions

Examples of organ-supporting botanicals

Treatment	Mechanism	Dose	Remarks
Panax ginseng [59–62]	Ginsenosides increase energy, increase vasodilation, improve blood flow, and support immune function.	250 mg once, twice, or three times a day	Is well tolerated but taken later in the day may be somewhat energizing for some people
Hippophae rhamnoides [58]	Broad-spectrum polyphenolic—Provides antioxidants, protects mitochondria, enhances vascular health.	500 mg of oil extract once or twice a day	50–100 ml of sea buckthorn juice per day is also rich in these compounds
Nigela sativa [63]	Increases acetylcholine in the brain and decreases inflammation including neuroinflammation.	1000 mg per day of black cumin seed oil	The seeds can be ground and eaten as well
Vinpocetine [56, 57]	Targets cyclic nucleotide phosphodiesterase 1 (PDE1) and decreases vascular inflammation.	10 mg once or twice per day	Absolutely contraindicated in pregnancy

Treatment	Mechanism	Dose	Remarks
Crocus sativa [53–55]	Crocusatins decrease neuroinflammation and support mood.	50 mg once or twice per day	Saffron can be consumed as a spice. Some products are prohibitively expensive and others are more accessible
Crataegus oxycantha [51, 52]	Flavone glycosides can recondition the vascular endothelium including the endothelial glycocalyx	500 mg once or twice per day 3 ml of tincture (water and ethanol extract) once or twice per day	Higher amounts are sometimes used early in treatment with patients who suffer from heart failure
Silymarin [46–50]	From *Silybum marianum*—Flavonolignans act as membrane stabilizers for cells, organelle, nucleus; increases glutathione levels	300 mg of milk thistle extract (80% silymarin) once or twice per day	Is useful for preventing ECM fibrosis; used for variety of hepatic issues, including NAFLD
Ginkgo biloba [43–45]	Flavonoids and terpenes stabilize the vascular endothelium; neuroprotective, cardio and renal protective	120 mg once or twice per day (standardized to 24% ginkgo flavoglycones and 6% terpenes)	May augment memory in those with cerebrovascular disease depending on level of dysfunction and damage
Colchicum autumnale [67–71]	Colchicine reduces inflammation and excessive matrix deposition in heart and kidney tissue. Reduces neutrophil extracellular traps in heart muscle post MI	Tincture of *Colchicum autumnale* 1 ml or 2 ml, twice or three times a day	In an acute care situation, colchicine (the pure alkaloid) is likely to be used

References

1. Lu P, Takai K, Weaver VM, Werb Z. Extracellular matrix degradation and remodeling in development and disease. Cold Spring Harb Perspect Biol. 2011;3(12):a005058.
2. Berdiaki A, Neagu M, Tzanakakis P, Spyridaki I, Pérez S, Nikitovic D. Extracellular matrix components and Mechanosensing pathways in health and disease. Biomol Ther. 2024;14(9):1186.
3. Taddei M, Giannoni E, Fiaschi T, Chiarugi P. Anoikis: an emerging hallmark in health and diseases. J Pathol. 2011;226(2):380–93.
4. Iozzo RV, Gubbiotti MA. Extracellular matrix: the driving force of mammalian diseases. Matrix Biol. 2018;71:1–9.
5. Panciera T, Azzolin L, Cordenonsi M, Piccolo S. Mechanobiology of YAP and TAZ in physiology and disease. Nat Rev Mol Cell Biol. 2017;18(12):758–70.
6. Liu S, Yao S, Yang H, Liu S, Wang Y. Autophagy: regulator of cell death. Cell Death Dis. 2023;14(10):648.
7. Schaefer L, Dikic I. Autophagy: instructions from the extracellular matrix. Matrix Biol. 2021;100-101:1–8.
8. Neill T, Schaefer L, Iozzo RV. Instructive roles of extracellular matrix on autophagy. Am J Pathol. 2014;184(8):2146–53.
9. Santinha D, et al. Remodeling of the cardiac extracellular matrix proteome during chronological and pathological aging. Mol Cell Proteomics. 2024;23(1):100706.
10. Aratani S, Nakanishi M. Recent advances in Senolysis for age-related diseases. Physiology. 2023;38(5):205–16.
11. Mebratu YA, Soni S, Rosas LE, Rojas M, Horowitz JC, Nho RS. The aged extracellular matrix and the profibrotic role of senescence-associated secretory phenotype. Am J Phys Cell Phys. 2023;325(3):C565–79.
12. Frangogiannis NG. The extracellular matrix in ischemic and nonischemic heart failure. Circ Res. 2019;125(1):117–46.
13. Freitas-Rodríguez S, Folgueras AR, López-Otín C. The role of matrix metalloproteinases in aging: tissue remodeling and beyond. Biochim et Biophys Acta (BBA) – Mol Cell Res. 2017;1864(11):2015–25.
14. Li L, He M, Tang X, Huang J, Li J, Hong X, et al. Proteomic landscape of the extracellular matrix in the fibrotic kidney. Kidney Int. 2023;103(6):1063–76.
15. Rayego-Mateos S, Campillo S, Rodrigues-Diez Raúl R, Tejera-Muñoz A, Marquez-Exposito L, Goldschmeding R, et al. Interplay between extracellular matrix components and cellular and molecular mechanisms in kidney fibrosis. Clin Sci. 2021;135(16):1999–2029.
16. Orvalho JS, Cowgill LD. Cardiorenal syndrome: diagnosis and management. Vet Clin N Am Small Anim Pract. 2017;47(5):1083–102.

17. Kercheva M, Ryabov V, Gombozhapova A, Stepanov I, Kzhyshkowska J. Macrophages of the Cardiorenal Axis and myocardial infarction. Biomedicines. 2023;11(7):1843.
18. Rangaswami J, Bhalla V, Blair JEA, Chang TI, Costa S, Lentine KL, et al. Cardiorenal syndrome: classification, pathophysiology, diagnosis, and treatment strategies: a scientific statement from the American Heart Association. Circulation. 2019;139(16)
19. Hiraiwa H, Okumura T, Murohara T. The cardiosplenic axis: the prognostic role of the spleen in heart failure. Heart Fail Rev. 2022;27(6):2005–15.
20. Ismahil MA, Hamid T, Bansal SS, Patel B, Kingery JR, Prabhu SD. Remodeling of the mononuclear phagocyte network underlies chronic inflammation and disease progression in heart failure: critical importance of the cardiosplenic axis. Circ Res. 2014;114(2):266–82.
21. Deng Z, Fear MW, Suk Choi Y, Wood FM, Allahham A, Mutsaers SE, et al. The extracellular matrix and mechanotransduction in pulmonary fibrosis. Int J Biochem Cell Biol. 2020;126:105802.
22. He M, Zhu H, Dong J, Lin W, Li B, Li Y, et al. Low-intensity pulsed ultrasound improves metabolic dysregulation in obese mice by suppressing inflammation and extracellular matrix remodeling. Ultrasonics. 2025;145:107488.
23. Bidan CM, Veldsink AC, Meurs H, Gosens R. Airway and extracellular matrix mechanics in COPD. Front Physiol. 2015;6
24. Horn P, Tacke F. Metabolic reprogramming in liver fibrosis. Cell Metab. 2024;36(7):1439–55.
25. Won SM, Oh KK, Gupta H, Ganesan R, Sharma SP, Jeong JJ, et al. The link between gut microbiota and hepatic encephalopathy. Int J Mol Sci. 2022;23(16):8999.
26. Albuquerque-Souza E, Sahingur SE. Periodontitis, chronic liver diseases, and the emerging oral-gut-liver axis. Periodontology. 2000;89(1):125–41.
27. Weissenborn K. Hepatic encephalopathy: definition, clinical grading and diagnostic principles. Drugs. 2019;79(S1):5–9.
28. Oey RC, van Buuren HR, de Man RA. The diagnostic work-up in patients with ascites: current guidelines and future prospects. Neth J Med. 2016;74(8):330–5.
29. Melouane A, Yoshioka M, St-Amand J. Extracellular matrix/mitochondria pathway: a novel potential target for sarcopenia. Mitochondrion. 2020;50:63–70.
30. Bonneh-Barkay D, Wiley CA. Brain extracellular matrix in neurodegeneration. Brain Pathol. 2009;19(4):573–85.
31. Jang DG, Sim HJ, Song EK, Kwon T, Park TJ. Extracellular matrixes and neuroinflammation. J Biochem Mol Biol. 2020;53(10):491–9.
32. Sun Y, Deng Y, Xiao M, Hu L, Li Z, Chen C. Chondroitin sulfate proteoglycans inhibit the migration and differentiation of oligodendrocyte precursor cells and its counteractive interaction with laminin. Int J Mol Med. 2017;40(6)

33. Lee IH. Mechanisms and disease implications of sirtuin-mediated autophagic regulation. Exp Mol Med. 2019;51(9):1–11.
34. Chung KW, Chung HY. The effects of calorie restriction on autophagy: role on aging intervention. Nutrients. 2019;11(12):2923.
35. Cui Z, Zhao X, Amevor FK, Du X, Wang Y, Li D, et al. Therapeutic application of quercetin in aging-related diseases: SIRT1 as a potential mechanism. Front Immunol. 2022;13
36. Hu F, Hu T, Qiao Y, Huang H, Zhang Z, Huang W, et al. Berberine inhibits excessive autophagy and protects myocardium against ischemia/reperfusion injury via the RhoE/AMPK pathway. Int J Mol Med. 2024;53(5)
37. Shan ZL. The effects of Astragalus Membranaceus active extracts on autophagy-related diseases. Int J Mol Sci. 2019;20(8):1904.
38. Madeo F, Bauer MA, Carmona-Gutierrez D, Kroemer G. Spermidine: a physiological autophagy inducer acting as an anti-aging vitamin in humans? Autophagy. 2018;15(1):165–8.
39. King KE, McCormick JJ, Kenny GP. Temperature-dependent relationship of autophagy and apoptotic signaling during cold-water immersion in young and older males. Adv Biol. 2024;8(3):e2300560.
40. Imb M, Véghelyi Z, Maurer M, Kühnel H. Exploring Senolytic and Senomorphic properties of medicinal plants for anti-aging therapies. Int J Mol Sci. 2024;25(19):10419.
41. Chaib S, Tchkonia T, Kirkland JL. Cellular senescence and senolytics: the path to the clinic. Nat Med. 2022;28(8):1556–68.
42. Liu X, Bian H, Dou QL, Huang XW, Tao WY, Liu WH, et al. Ginkgetin alleviates inflammation, oxidative stress, and apoptosis induced by hypoxia/Reoxygenation in H9C2 cells via Caspase-3 dependent pathway. Biomed Res Int. 2020;2020:1–9.
43. Liu Y, Niu P, Yan J, Ji H, Wang Z, Jin X, et al. Efficacy and safety of Ginkgo biloba extract in the treatment of unstable angina pectoris: a systematic review and network meta-analysis. J Ethnopharmacol. 2024;331:118297.
44. Singh SK, Srivastav S, Castellani RJ, Plascencia-Villa G, Perry G. Neuroprotective and antioxidant effect of Ginkgo biloba extract against AD and other neurological disorders. Neurotherapeutics. 2019;16(3):666–74.
45. Han J, Pang X, Shi X, Zhang Y, Peng Z, Xing Y. Ginkgo biloba extract EGB761 ameliorates the extracellular matrix accumulation and mesenchymal transformation of renal tubules in diabetic kidney disease by inhibiting endoplasmic reticulum stress. Abu Shahin N, editor. Biomed Res Int. 2021;2021:1–11.
46. Aghemo A, Alekseeva OP, Angelico F, Bakulin IG, Bakulina NV, Bordin D, et al. Role of silymarin as antioxidant in clinical management of chronic liver diseases: a narrative review. Ann Med. 2022;54(1):1548–60.
47. Federico A, Dallio M, Loguercio C. Silymarin/Silybin and chronic liver disease: a marriage of many years. Molecules. 2017;22(2):191.

48. Dluholucký S, Snitková M, Knapková M, Cibirová M, Mydlová Z. Results of diagnostics and treatment of amanita phalloides poisoning in Slovakia (2004–2020). Toxicon. 2022;219:106927.
49. Gillessen A, Angelico F, Chen J, Lu L, Lucena MI, Fu Q, et al. Silymarin for treating toxic liver disease: international consensus recommendations. Gastro Hep Advances. 2022;1(5):882–93.
50. Momeni A. Effect of Silymarin in the prevention of cisplatin nephrotoxicity, a clinical trial study. J Clin Diagn Res. 2015;9(4)
51. Furey A, Tassell M, Kingston R, Gilroy D, Lehane M. Hawthorn (Crataegus spp.) in the treatment of cardiovascular disease. Pharmacogn Rev. 2010;4(7):32.
52. Zorniak M, Szydlo B, Krzeminski TF. Crataegus special extract WS 1442: up-to-date review of experimental and clinical experiences. J Physiol Pharmacol. 2017;68(4):521–6.
53. Khazdair MR, Boskabady MH, Hosseini M, Rezaee R, Tsatsakis M. The effects of Crocus sativus (saffron) and its constituents on nervous system: a review. Avicenna J Phytomed. 2015;5(5):376–91.
54. Wani A, Al Rihani SB, Sharma A, Weadick B, Govindarajan R, Khan SU, et al. Crocetin promotes clearance of amyloid-β by inducing autophagy via the STK11/LKB1-mediated AMPK pathway. Autophagy. 2021;17(11):3813–32.
55. Hatziagapiou K, Kakouri E, Lambrou GI, Bethanis K, Tarantilis PA. Antioxidant properties of crocus Sativus L. and its constituents and relevance to neurodegenerative diseases; focus on Alzheimer's and Parkinson's disease. Curr Neuropharmacol. 2019;17(4):377–402.
56. Panda PK, Ramachandran A, Panda P, Sharawat IK. Safety and efficacy of Vinpocetine as a neuroprotective agent in acute ischemic stroke: a systematic review and meta-analysis. Neurocrit Care. 2022;37(1):314–25.
57. Zhang Y, Li J, Yan C. An update on Vinpocetine: new discoveries and clinical implications. Eur J Pharmacol. 2018;819:30–4.
58. Żuchowski J. Phytochemistry and pharmacology of sea buckthorn (Elaeagnus rhamnoides; syn. Hippophae rhamnoides): progress from 2010 to 2021. Phytochem Rev Proc Phytochem Soc Europe. 2022;22(1):1–31.
59. Irfan M, Kwak YS, Han CK, Hyun SH, Rhee MH. Adaptogenic effects of Panax ginseng on modulation of cardiovascular functions. J Ginseng Res. 2020;44(4)
60. Cao X, Yao F, Zhang B, Sun X. Mitochondrial dysfunction in heart diseases: potential therapeutic effects of *Panax ginseng*. Front Pharmacol. 2023;14:1218803.
61. Lee SY. Anti-metastatic and anti-inflammatory effects of matrix metalloproteinase inhibition by Ginsenosides. Biomedicines. 2021;9(2):198.
62. Im DS. Pro-resolving effect of Ginsenosides as an anti-inflammatory mechanism of Panax ginseng. Biomol Ther. 2020;10(3):444.

63. Hannan MA, Rahman MA, Sohag AAM, Uddin MJ, Dash R, Sikder MH, et al. Black cumin (Nigella sativa L.): a comprehensive review on Phytochemistry, health benefits, molecular pharmacology, and safety. Nutrients. 2021;13(6):1784.
64. Dalli M, Bekkouch O, Azizi S, Azghar A, Gseyra N, Kim B. Nigella sativa L. Phytochemistry and pharmacological activities: a review (2019–2021). Biomol Ther. 2021;12(1):20.
65. Donyavi V, Rafiee Zadeh A, Foroughi Eghbal A, Mirghazanfari S, Ghasemzadeh M, Nassireslami E. *Nigella sativa* extract in the treatment of depression and serum brain-derived neurotrophic factor (BDNF) levels. J Res Med Sci. 2022;27(1):28.
66. Gawas CG, Mathur S, Wani M, Tabassum H. *Nigella sativa* and its nano-mediated approach toward management of neurodegenerative disorders: a review. Ibrain. 2023;9(1):111–23.
67. Li JJ, Lee SH, Kim DK, Jin R, Jung DS, Kwak SJ, et al. Colchicine attenuates inflammatory cell infiltration and extracellular matrix accumulation in diabetic nephropathy. AJP Renal Physiol. 2009;297(1):F200–9.
68. Huang W, Sun H, Pan X, Fei L, Guo M, Bao H, et al. Effects of colchicine on synthesis and excretion of cytokines and extracellular matrix by human renal fibroblasts. Chin J Pediatr. 2004;42(7):524–8.
69. Vaidya K, Tucker B, Kurup R, Khandkar C, Pandzic E, Barraclough J, et al. Colchicine inhibits neutrophil extracellular trap formation in patients with acute coronary syndrome after percutaneous coronary intervention. J Am Heart Assoc. 2021;10(1)
70. Bouabdallaoui N, Tardif JC, Waters DD, Pinto FJ, Maggioni AP, Diaz R, et al. Time-to-treatment initiation of colchicine and cardiovascular outcomes after myocardial infarction in the colchicine cardiovascular outcomes trial (COLCOT). Eur Heart J. 2020;41(42):4092–9.
71. Yousefzadeh MJ, Zhu Y, McGowan SJ, Angelini L, Fuhrmann-Stroissnigg H, Xu M, et al. Fisetin is a senotherapeutic that extends health and lifespan. EBioMedicine. 2018;36:18–28.

Neoplasm: Examples of Extracellular Matrix Involvement and Treatment

12

Cancer, the clinical term for various neoplasms, is the second leading cause of death globally and in the United States. Successful treatment has gradually improved due to massive research efforts. Survivorship was 49% in the mid-1970s and is now about 68%. Some cancers are much more survivable with treatment than others [1]. For example, pancreatic cancer has about a 5% five-year survival rate, whereas thyroid cancer has about a 98% survival rate. Advances in molecular biology and genetics have increased the understanding of cancer. This includes the science of cancer genetics, interaction with the immune system, tumor vulnerabilities, and the critical events in the tumor microenvironment. New biomedical techniques exist such as the use of monoclonal antibodies to target tumors and draw the immune system to recognize and attack them. Cytotoxic therapies that target hyperproliferative cells remain the mainstay of treatment.

Some of the emerging knowledge about the tumor microenvironment is the basis of this chapter, that is, the events in the extracellular matrix in the progression of cancer.

Cancer starts with a mutation, particularly of the genes that are related to the cellular growth control [2]. These proto-oncogenes can fulfill normal functions, but upon mutation and overexpression, they can convert to what are called oncogenes. Cancer is also evidenced by failures of tumor suppressor genes, such as TP53, which ought to cause a cell on the developmental road to cancer

F. Smith, *The Extracellular Matrix in Health and Disease*,
https://doi.org/10.1007/978-3-031-94465-9_12

to undergo apoptosis. DNA repair genes can sometimes fix mutations (Fig. 12.1).

Mutations typically become more likely with age, with observable chromosomal changes such as the Philadelphia chromosome, a translocation between chromosomes 9 and 22, and subsequent fusion of genes. Some mutations are inherited, such as faulty DNA repair genes BRCA1 and BRCA2. The causes of mutation can range from random events—mistakes in chromosome replication—to physical or energetic agents such as ultraviolet light or carcinogenic compounds from the environment and diet [3].

Mutations caused by carcinogenic factors can often be blocked by endogenous or nutritional antioxidants. Some mutations can be rectified, such as when pyrimidine dimers caused by photodimerization (UV light) are fixed by nucleotide excision repair enzymes. Persistent mutations can lead to progressive change of a cell to a cancer type. It may start to divide more frequently than normal. Under a microscope, it may take on appearances that look less mature, which is a process that can result in anaplasia. The cell might start to change its alignment inside of its tissue, literally not fitting into surrounding structures. This is the stage of promotion and can last for decades. When that cell, should it survive apop-

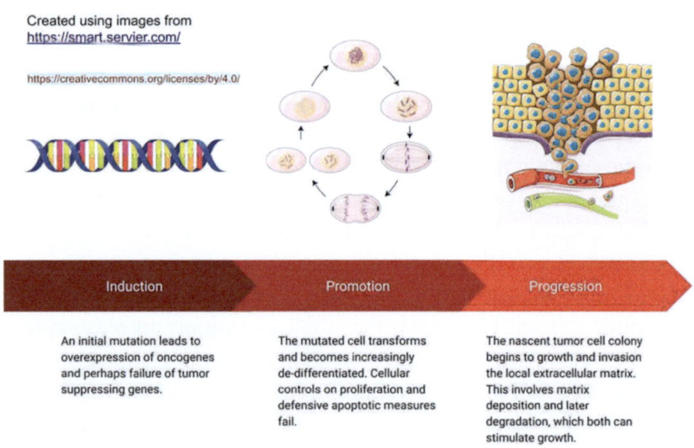

Fig. 12.1 Cancer process

totic failsafe, arrives at a cell type that has the hallmarks of a cancer cell, it will now attempt to forge ahead through its surrounding tissues and vastly replicate itself. At this point, the battle of a parasitic and hostile neoplastic cell, and the body, is fought within the extracellular matrix.

The discussion in this chapter centers on the ECM. Cancer is a multifactorial and complex disease, but the ECM is a pivotal area of the success, or hopefully failure, of a neoplastic colony of cells to gain a foothold and spread. The relevance to naturopathic medicine is twofold. On the one hand, there are natural substances, particularly plant extracts, that can frustrate many of the strategies that cancer cells use to invade and dominate the ECM. But it is also important to bear in mind that the health of the ECM, or its dysfunction as described in preceding chapters, can set the stage for that success or failure. An oxidized, stiff ECM that induces senescent behavior in cells and inhibits autophagy presents a better environment for many cancers. In a 2023 review, Liang et al. lay out the stages of cancer invasion and domination of the microenvironment. In this article, they bring great clarity to this complex process and provide a model whereby plant extracts can be understood to be potentially effective.

Early Phases: Deposition of Additional Matrix

When a neoplastic mass is beginning to gain numbers and then spread locally, it first creates excess ECM, particularly collagen, around itself [4]. If this is ECM near a basement membrane, the collagen production will be centered beyond the basement membrane that was breached by the cancer cell mass. This collagen is secreted by fibroblasts, which do so under the influence of cytokines. This exuberant collagen production is often accompanied by differentiation into myofibroblasts.

This collagen has a dual purpose. Externally, it provides some cover from circulating natural killer cells, which might attack the nascent cancer. Internally, it provides a type of mechanotransduction signal that can increase cancer cell proliferation. The increased stiffness of abundant crosslinked (covalently) collagen, via fibronectin–integrin connections, can have an increase in mitosis as an effect [5]. This positive feedback effect is created by the cancer cells themselves.

At the leading edge of this collagen front is a specialized podocyte created by the neoplastic cells. It has a core of actin fibrils and is coated with matrix metalloproteinases. This "invasdasome" will start to tunnel into the surrounding ECM. This creates room for more cancer cells [6]. It adds to a strategy of matrix destruction that is critical to the success of the neoplastic colony. (Fig. 12.2).

Cancer cells can gain control of fibroblasts [7] (as noted), as well as macrophages and neutrophils [8–10]. Cancer-associated macrophages will secrete matrix metalloproteinases, as can cancer-associated fibroblasts, influenced by cancer cell secretion of integrins. [11] Additional proteases and elastases will

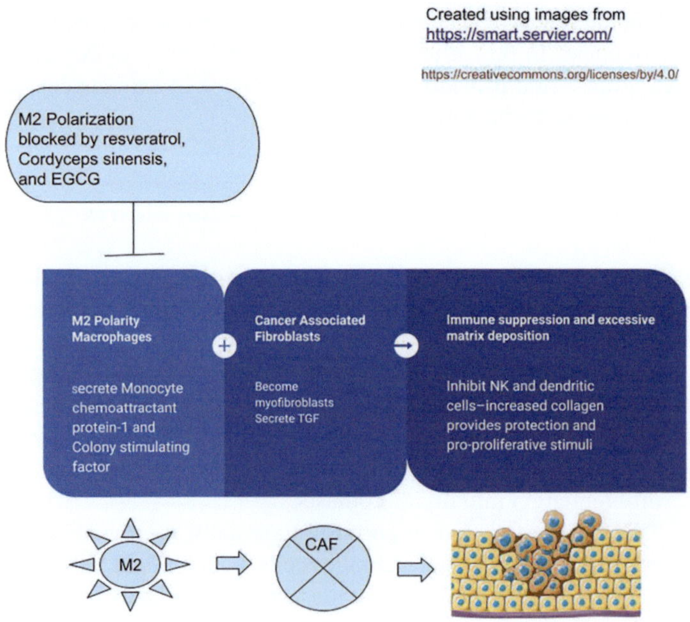

Fig. 12.2 M2 polarity

eventually be released by cancer-associated neutrophils. This can facilitate tumor spread and also cause the digestion of laminins, which results in basement membrane destruction. The damaged fragments of the ECM provoke inflammation and are themselves sources of energy, a kind of food, for neoplastic cells. The damage of the ECM protein scaffolding has another purpose. The vesicles attached to the ECM contain important growth factors, such as vegetative endothelial growth factor (VEGF) and platelet-derived growth factor (PDGF). [12] These compounds are never meant to be all liberated at the same time. When cancer-associated cells essentially release these vesicles and their contents, it has an angiogenic effect. More angiogenesis, with sprouting of blood vessels in the vicinity of the tumor, provides a more robust blood supply. This not only brings oxygen and nutrients to the cancer cells, but creates more opportunities for metastasis. (Fig. 12.3).

The neoplastic mass can convert some epithelial tissues to mesenchyme, a multipotent tissue that can redevelop into different forms [13]. In this case, the mesenchymal development will

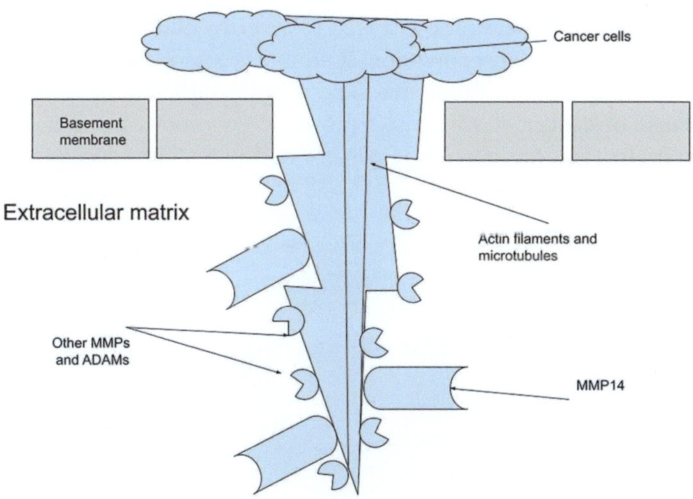

Fig. 12.3 Invadosome

turn to the creation of myofibroblasts. The increase of local TGF-beta from these myofibroblasts has an inhibitory effect on both natural killer cells and dendritic cells. NK cells are critical aspects of innate immune responses to the cancer cells. Dendritic cells are key antigen-presenting cells (APC), so the ability of cancer cells to silence some of the local APC has an inhibiting effect on adaptive immune responses. Cancer-associated fibroblasts also secreted certain integrins, which can assist cells in invading the surrounding tissues (Fig. 12.4). A certain integrin, alpha11Beta1, can make ECM particularly stiffer, which is beneficial to cancer cells.

The impact of an inflammatory phenotype on cancer opportunism is becoming better understood. The tumor suppressor protein, p53, is less active under conditions of high NFkB due to downregulation of expression of TP53 gene [14]. Inflammation leads to reactive stiffening of the matrix, which can, through mechanotransduction, have a proliferative effect on cancer cells. The process of senolysis, as described in the previous chapter, is important for preventing the development of a senescence-associated secretory phenotype [15]. This stage of chronic inflammation, accumulation of advanced glycemic end products, and elevated oxidative stress will lead to an extracellular matrix that promotes oncogene expression. It promotes angiogenesis and cellular proliferation. While this state is not a sufficient or solitary cause of cancer, it will create favorable conditions for mutated cells to start the neoplastic project and potentially succeed in overcoming host defenses.

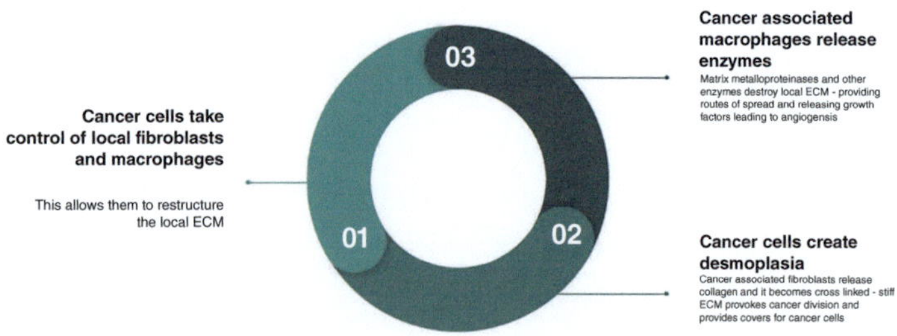

Fig. 12.4 Cancer steps in ECM

Natural Substances That Can Discourage Collagen Deposition Around the Cancer Cells

Cancer-associated fibroblasts, under the influence of transforming growth factor beta (TGFb), will deposit large amounts of collagen near the neoplastic cells. Increased lysyl oxidase activity will crosslink this collagen, increasing the stiffness. Certain plant extracts will inhibit both excessive collagen production as well as the alternation of the biochemistry of the ECM that results in a more crosslinked version of the (overabundant) collagen, and a stiffer matrix that supports tumor development. The degree to which this inhibition can happen clinically, the true magnitude of effect, is not known, but given the safety and the multiple benefits of these plant extracts, including a general anti-inflammatory effect, their use seems justified.

Gingketin is a flavonoid from *Ginkgo biloba* and has been found to inhibit excess matrix production, including deposition of collagen IV, fibronectin, and laminin. [4, 15] This appears to work by inhibiting AMPK and mTOR. Isoliquiritigenin from *Glycyrrhiza glabra* (licorice) can also decrease local inflammation and collagen deposition [4]. In general, many of the phytochemical antifibrotics discussed in this book are applicable here. In this case, the desmoplasia that is discouraged by these polyphenols is not an overreaction to injury, but a strategy of a neoplasm to subdue, and then spread through, the ECM. Thymoquinone, from *Nigella sativa*, can prevent excessive collagen deposition by inhibiting its mRNA expression, and by phosphorylating AMPK in the fibroblasts, which leads to less protein (collagen) synthesis [16].

Asiatic acid from *Centella asiatica* is a suppressor of TGF-beta. The herb *C. asiatica* is known to be useful for wound healing and preventing scar formation [17].

Silibinin is a flavonoid from *Silybum marianum* (milk thistle) and has been shown to inhibit the action of integrin in assisting cancer cells to migrate along actin filaments. Neoplastic cells can release integrin into the ECM, which has several effects and can also be used in the migration of those cancer cells [18].

Preventing Excessive ECM Degradation

Natural substances can prevent destruction of the ECM and vesicle release of VEGF and PDGF. Some of these compounds can also prevent excessive deposition, such that they have a regulating effect on both overproduction and crosslinking of collagen and on the excessive activation of MMPs and subsequent degradation of the ECM [19].

Artemisinin, from plants such as *Artemisia annua* (sweet wormwood), can inhibit activation of MMP-9, one of the key metalloproteinases that are activated by cancer cells [19].

Astragaloside IV, from *Astragalus membranaceous*, can increase the production of tissue inhibitor of metalloproteinases (TIMP-1), which controls excessive MMP activity [4].

Kaempferol is a flavonoid with many food sources such as capers, kale, brussels sprouts, apples, ginger, cabbage, cilantro, grapes, pumpkin, broccoli, leeks, and notably, saffron. Botanical herbs that contain kaempferol include *Hippophae rhamnoides*, *Rosmarinus officinalis*, and *Aloe vera*. It can inhibit degradation of collagen by proteases MMP-1, MMP-3, and MMP-13 [19, 20].

Berberine, an alkaloid from plants such as *Hydrastis canadensis*, can both inhibit MMP and at the same time prevent excessive collagen formation. It also inhibits Insulin-like growth factor 1 receptor, which is used by cancer cells to suppress apoptosis [21].

Reseveratrol has a dual effect of both reducing the mRNA levels of fibronectin and collagen, but also inhibits MMP-3, MMP-9, as well as lowering VEGF (an angiogenesis signal). Resveratrol also inhibits the activation of STAT3 signaling and reduces the percentage of M2-like macrophages [22].

Normalizing Resident ECM Macrophages Out of M2 Phenotype

Cancer cells can cause phenotype switching of resident macrophages from M1 to M2. This leads to less immune activation and more fibrosis. Although the M2 phenotype is important in healing and resolution of inflammation, when cancer cells push an M2 polarity, it begins to silence local immune responses. Moreover, the M2 macrophages encourage fibroblasts to convert to myofibroblasts by secreting monocyte chemoattractant protein-1 and colony-stimulating factor. This in turns leads (via TGF secretion) fibroblasts to become cancer-associated fibroblasts, which release more collagen and fibronectin, enhancing cancer invasiveness. Resveratol can inhibit this M2 polarity and has the added benefits of reducing TGF-β1 and IL-10, which are immune suppressing, but can also increase TNF-α and IFN-γ, which can help rally the immune system [4, 22]. Epigallocatechin gallate (EGCG) can also inhibit the M2 polarity, and similarly to resveratrol, can decrease TGF and increase TNF-alpha [23].

Interrupting Signals to Cancer-Associated Fibroblasts

Breaking Connections to TAM, TAF, and TAN

Curcuma longa, or turmeric, is used as a culinary herb across the world. Curcuminoids are linear diarylheptanoids and collectively are referred to as curcumin. This substance has multiple targets that inhibit the cancer process. It can be difficult to absorb, and some forms are phosphatidylcholine bound, and more recently, nanoparticles. The challenge is absorption from the gut but also delivery to the cell. In this case, the cell is a fibroblast in the ECM. Curcumin can prevent cancer-associated fibroblasts from secreting TGF-beta to the point that there is epithelial to mesenchymal transition. It also reduces IL-6 (a proinflammatory cytokine) and overall oxidative stress. It appears to block the mTOR pathway [4, 24, 25].

Natural Substances That Can Reactivate Immune System

There are many immunomodulatory substances in naturopathic medicine. In this section, the focus is on some examples that can help to reverse the localized suppression of immune response in the ECM wrought by cancer (Fig. 12.5).

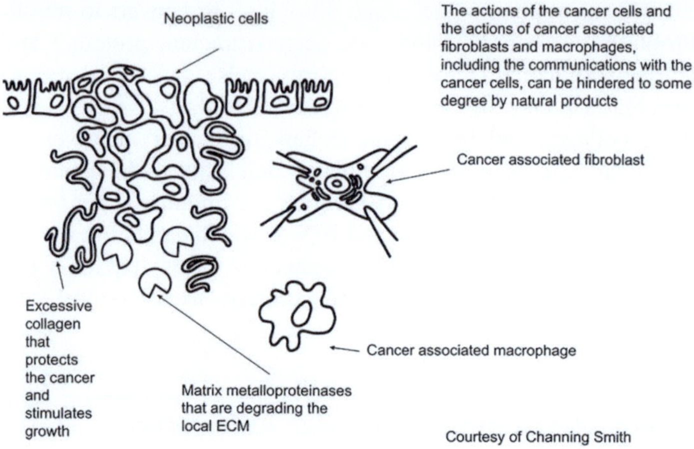

Fig. 12.5 Tumor microenvironment

Medicinal fungi are a very powerful arm of natural products, knowledge of which is increasing rapidly. *Grifola frondosa* (Maitake), *Lentinula edodes* (Shitake), and *Trametes versicolor* (Turkey tail) can increase natural killer cell activity. These mushrooms include a variety of compounds, including but not exclusively polysaccharides. These include beta-glucans, which can be processed by dendritic cells and cause multiple immune effects, often upregulating. They may also increase dendritic cell autophagy [26–28].

Plant compounds to reduce desmoplasia

Compound and example of source	Mechanism	Dose	Remarks
Gingketin from *Ginkgo biloba* [4]	Inhibiting AMPK and mTOR	*Ginkgo biloba* extract .80 mg two or three times per day (24% total ginkgo flavone glycosides, 6% total terpenes—Ginkgolides)	Ginkgo has other antioxidant effects

Compound and example of source	Mechanism	Dose	Remarks
Isoliquiritigenin from *Glycyrrhiza glabra* [4]	Decrease local inflammation	300 of *Glycyrrhiza* root extract once per day	Moderate doses are tolerable but higher doses can increase blood pressure due to increased aldosterone—Deglycyrrhizinated licorice avoids this effect and can be used as an alternate
Thymoquinone, from *Nigella sativa* [16]	Prevents excessive collagen deposition by inhibiting its mRNA expression, and by phosphorylating AMPK in the fibroblasts	Black cumin seed extract 400 mg once per day	*Nigella sativa* is the primary course of this compound General anti-inflammatory and antioxidant effects
Asiatic acid from *Centella asiatica* [17]	Inhibit TGF-beta	500 mg of *Centella asiatica* (Gotu kola) twice per day Or, 3 ml of tincture (water–ethanol extract) twice per day	Has wound-healing properties—Broad antifibrotic effects
Silibinin from *Silybum marianum* (milk thistle) [18]	Reduce integrin released by cancer-associated fibroblasts	250 mg milk thistle extract (80% silymarin) once per day	Has hepatoprotective and renal protective functions

These substances could be useful in preventing ECM fibrosis in non-neoplastic situations

Plant compounds to resist excess matrix degradation

Compounds and source	Mechanism	Dose	Remarks
Artemisinin, from *Artemisia annua* [19]	Inhibits MMP-9	500 mg twice per day	Has digestive support properties and anti-parasitic actions
Astragaloside IV, from *Astragalus membranaceous* [4]	Promotes tissue inhibitor of metalloproteinase	500 mg three times a day 3 ml of tincture (water–ethanol extract) three times a day	Has multiple effects on immune upregulation and the herb is an adaptogen
Kaempferol from *Rosmarinus officinale*, Aloe vera and multiple foods [20]	Inhibit degradation of collagen by proteases MMP-1, MMP-3, and MMP-13	500 mg of *Rosmarinus officinalis* twice per day	Found in capers, kale, Brussels sprouts, apples, ginger, cabbage, cilantro, grapes, pumpkin, broccoli, leeks, and saffron
Berberine, an alkaloid from plants such as *Hydrastis canadensis* [21]	Inhibits MMP9 but also inhibits excessive collagen formation	Berberine 500 mg twice per day	Aksi found in *Mahonia vulgaris, Mahonia aquifolium,* and *Coptis chinensis* Helps with insulin resistance Inhibits AMPK and is antifibrotic
Resveratrol [29]	Reduces excess fibronectin and collagen; lowers MMP-3, MMP-9, and VEGF	40 mg once a day or twice a day	Founds in grapes, dark chocolate, berries, peanuts, and red wine

Compounds to resist cancer control of fibroblasts and macrophages

Resveratrol [22]	Shift macrophage polarity to M1 and increase IFN-y and TNF-a secretion and by polarity switch, decrease TGF-β1 and IL-10	40 mg once a day or twice a day	Founds in grapes, dark chocolate, berries, peanuts, and red wine As noted above, has antifibrotic effects (multiple regulating actions on the ECM)
EGCG (epigallocatechin gallate) [23]	Shift macrophages to M1 polarity—Decrease TGF and increase TNF-a	200 mg EGCG once per day	Green tea and white tea contain this polyphenolic Apples, cocoa, pears, and chocolate also have EGCG as does (in lesser amounts) black tea
Cordyceps sinensis (a mushroom—Caterpillar fungus)	Causes M2 to M1 switch via binding to MAPK	500 mg Cordyceps three times a day	Standardized extracts might guarantee minimal glucans and polysaccharides and cordycepin, which is 3′-deoxyadenosine
Curcuma longa (Curcuminoids)	Reduces TGF-beta secretion and eIL-6 via inhibition of the mTOR pathway	Curcumin 500 mg twice per day(standardized to contain 95% curcuminoids)	Turmeric has lower yield but does contain these compounds—Better absorbed with fats. Phytosomes and nanoparticles can further enhance absorption and dispersal through the body

Strategies to support dendritic cell and natural killer cell function [26–28]

Compound and source	Mechanism	Dose	Remarks
Grifola frondosa (Maitake)	D fraction glucans activate dendritic cells and can mobilize NK cells	500 mg twice per day	Mushrooms are sometimes studied for one compound but in fact have an entourage of helpful compounds in them
Lentinula edodes (shiitake mushroom)	Mobilize NK cells—Contains terpenoids as well as glucans.	400 mg per day	The mushroom can be eaten in salads, soups, and stir frys
Trametes versicolor	Mobilizes NK cells via polysaccharide peptide (PSP) and polysaccharide krestin (PSK)	1000 mg twice per day	Also reduces inflammation

Key dietary considerations for ECM and cancer

Dietary consideration	Mechanism	Frequency	Remarks
Restrict added sugars [30–32]	Cancer cells will use sugars for anaerobic metabolism.	Keep added sugars below 10 g per day	Patient should not have an excessive carbohydrate load
Consume an anti-inflammatory fatty acid profile [33]	Changes eicosanoid and prostanoid profile to reduce inflammation. The secretory inflammatory phenotype is encouraging to cancer.	Daily fatty acids should keep omega 3 s at a ratio of 1–4 but even 1–6	Avoiding seed oils, trans fats and heated oils, and eating raw nuts, wheat germ, fish/seafood, and flax will help with omega-3 intake
Fruits and vegetables [34]	Provides nutrients such as vitamins A and C, but also flavonoids and polyphenols.	At least 10 servings a day of fruits and vegetables are needed	Phytochemicals from the plate are the foundation of nutritional support

Dietary consideration	Mechanism	Frequency	Remarks
Fermented foods [35]	Sources of probiotics, and prebiotics—Leads to a less inflammatory gut flora and healthier gut epithelium [35].	Several servings a day of fermented foods such as yogurt, sauerkraut, buttermilk, kim chi, miso, tempeh, kefir, etc.	A wide variety of ferments from different culinary traditions make these vital cultures easy to find

References

1. National Cancer Institute. Statistics, Graphs and Definitions | Division of Cancer Control and Population Sciences (DCCPS). cancercontrol.cancer.gov. 2022. Available from: https://cancercontrol.cancer.gov/ocs/statistics
2. de Visser KE, Joyce JA. The evolving tumor microenvironment: from cancer initiation to metastatic outgrowth. Cancer Cell. 2023;41(3):374–403.
3. Ostroverkhova D, Przytycka TM, Panchenko AR. Cancer driver mutations: predictions and reality. Trends Mol Med. 2023;29(7)
4. Liang D, Liu L, Zhao Y, Luo Z, He Y, Li Y, et al. Targeting extracellular matrix through phytochemicals: a promising approach of multi-step actions on the treatment and prevention of cancer. Front Pharmacol. 2023;14
5. Marozzi M, Parnigoni A, Negri A, Viola M, Vigetti D, Passi A, et al. Inflammation, extracellular matrix remodeling, and proteostasis in tumor microenvironment. Int J Mol Sci. 2021;22(15):8102.
6. Augoff K, Hryniewicz-Jankowska A, Tabola R. Invadopodia: clearing the way for cancer cell invasion. Ann Transl Med. 2020;8(14)
7. Biffi G, Tuveson DA. Diversity and biology of cancer-associated fibroblasts. Physiol Rev. 2021;101(1):147–76.
8. Pan Y, Yu Y, Wang X, Zhang T. Tumor-associated macrophages in tumor immunity. Front Immunol. 2020;11
9. Varol C, Sagi I. Phagocyte – extracellular matrix crosstalk empowers tumor development and dissemination. FEBS J. 2017;285(4):734–51.
10. Mehta AK, Kadel S, Townsend MG, Oliwa M, Guerriero JL. Macrophage biology and mechanisms of immune suppression in breast cancer. Front Immunol. 2021;12

11. Huang H. Matrix metalloproteinase-9 (MMP-9) as a cancer biomarker and MMP-9 biosensors: recent advances. Sensors. 2018;18(10):3249.
12. Chang WH, Cerione RA, Antonyak MA. Extracellular vesicles and their roles in cancer progression. Methods Mol Biol. 2021;2174:143–70.
13. Du F, Li J, Zhong X, Zhang Z, Zhao Y. Endothelial-to-mesenchymal transition in the tumor microenvironment: roles of transforming growth factor-β and matrix metalloproteins. Heliyon. 2024;10(21):e40118.
14. Carrà G, Lingua MF, Maffeo B, Taulli R, Morotti A. P53 vs NF-κB: the role of nuclear factor-kappa B in the regulation of p53 activity and vice versa. Cell Mol Life Sci. 2020;77(22):4449–58.
15. Wei L, Jian P, Erjiong H, Qihan Z. Ginkgetin alleviates high glucose-evoked mesangial cell oxidative stress injury, inflammation, and extracellular matrix (ECM) deposition in an AMPK/mTOR-mediated autophagy axis. Chem Biol Drug Des. 2021;98(4):620–30.
16. Khan MA, Tania M, Fu J. Epigenetic role of thymoquinone: impact on cellular mechanism and cancer therapeutics. Drug Discov Today. 2019;24(12):2315–22.
17. Cui Q, Ren J, Zhou Q, Yang Q, Li B. Effect of asiatic acid on epithelial-mesenchymal transition of human alveolar epithelium A549 cells induced by TGF-β1. Oncol Lett. 2019;17(5)
18. Deep G, Kumar R, Jain AK, Agarwal C, Agarwal R. Silibinin inhibits fibronectin induced motility, invasiveness and survival in human prostate carcinoma PC3 cells via targeting integrin signaling. Mutat Res. 2014;768:35–46.
19. Islam MT, Jang NH, Lee HJ. Natural products as regulators against matrix metalloproteinases for the treatment of cancer. Biomedicines. 2024;12(4):794.
20. Periferakis A, Periferakis K, Badarau IA, Petran EM, Popa DC, Caruntu A, et al. Kaempferol: antimicrobial properties, sources, clinical, and traditional applications. Int J Mol Sci. 2022;23(23):15054.
21. Lin JP, Yang JS, Wu CC, Lin SS, Hsieh WT, Lin ML, et al. Berberine induced down-regulation of matrix metalloproteinase-1, −2 and −9 in human gastric cancer cells (SNU-5) in vitro. In vivo (Athens, Greece). 2008;22(2):223–30.
22. Talib WH, Alsayed AR, Farhan F, Al Kury LT. Resveratrol and tumor microenvironment: mechanistic basis and therapeutic targets. Molecules (Basel, Switzerland). 2020;25(18):E4282.
23. Li D, Cao D, Sun Y, Cui Y, Zhang Y, Jiang J, et al. The roles of epigallocatechin gallate in the tumor microenvironment, metabolic reprogramming, and immunotherapy. Front Immunol. 2024:15.
24. Liu H, Liu A, Shi C, Li B. Curcumin suppresses transforming growth factor-β1-induced cardiac fibroblast differentiation via inhibition of Smad-2 and p38 MAPK signaling pathways. Exp Ther Med. 2016;11(3):998–1004.

25. Du Y, Long Q, Zhang L, Shi Y, Liu X, Li X, et al. Curcumin inhibits cancer-associated fibroblast-driven prostate cancer invasion through MAOA/mTOR/HIF-1α signaling. Int J Oncol. 2015;47(6):2064–72.
26. Hetland G, Tangen JM, Mahmood F, Mirlashari MR, Nissen-Meyer LSH, Nentwich I, et al. Antitumor, anti-inflammatory and Antiallergic effects of Agaricus blazei mushroom extract and the related medicinal basidiomycetes mushrooms, Hericium erinaceus and Grifola frondosa: a review of preclinical and clinical studies. Nutrients. 2020;12(5):1339.
27. Park HJ. Current uses of mushrooms in cancer treatment and their anticancer mechanisms. Int J Mol Sci. 2022;23(18):10502.
28. Mishra V, Tripathi V, Yadav P, Singh MP. Beta glucan as an immune stimulant in tumor microenvironment – insight into lessons and promises from past decade. Int J Biol Macromol. 2023;234:123617.
29. Sun Y, Zhou QM, Lu YY, Zhang H, Chen QL, Zhao M, et al. Resveratrol inhibits the migration and metastasis of MDA-MB-231 human breast cancer by reversing TGF-β1-induced epithelial-mesenchymal transition. Molecules. 2019;24(6):1131.
30. Debras C, Chazelas E, Srour B, Kesse-Guyot E, Julia C, Zelek L, et al. Total and added sugar intakes, sugar types, and cancer risk: results from the prospective NutriNet-santé cohort. Am J Clin Nutr. 2020;112(5):1267–79.
31. Vaupel P, Schmidberger H, Mayer A. The Warburg effect: essential part of metabolic reprogramming and central contributor to cancer progression. Int J Radiat Biol. 2019;95(7):912–9.
32. Vaupel P, Multhoff G. Revisiting the Warburg effect: historical dogma versus current understanding. J Physiol. 2021;599(6):1745–57.
33. Djuricic I, Calder PC. Beneficial outcomes of Omega-6 and Omega-3 polyunsaturated fatty acids on human health: an update for 2021. Nutrients. 2021;13(7):2421.
34. Hardt L, Mahamat-Saleh Y, Aune D, Schlesinger S. Plant-based diets and cancer prognosis: a review of recent research. Curr Nutr Rep. 2022;11(4)
35. Cuamatzin-García L, Rodríguez-Rugarcía P, El-Kassis EG, Galicia G, et al. Traditional fermented foods and beverages from around the world and their health benefits. Microorganisms. 2022;10(6):1151.

Index

F. Smith, *The Extracellular Matrix in Health and Disease*,
https://doi.org/10.1007/978-3-031-94465-9